BIOCHEMISTRY OF THE RETINA

1st International Symposium on the Biochemistry
of the Retina, London, September 1964

BIOCHEMISTRY OF THE RETINA

Edited by

Clive N Graymore

Institute of Ophthalmology, University of London, England

Supplement to Experimental Eye Research

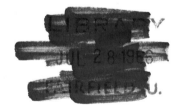

1965
Academic Press
London and New York

ACADEMIC PRESS INC. (LONDON) LTD
Berkeley Square House
Berkeley Square
London, W.1.

U.S. Edition published by
ACADEMIC PRESS INC.
111 Fifth Avenue
New York, New York 10003

Library of Congress Catalog Card Number: 65–27549

PRINTED IN GREAT BRITAIN BY
WILLMER BROTHERS LIMITED, BIRKENHEAD

Foreword

The body interprets much of its environment through two fragile tissue entities weighing scarcely more than 100 mg apiece. To determine their molecular architecture, the nature and distribution of the complex enzyme sequences they contain, and to clarify the function of the individual layers presents an exciting challenge. To understand the deviations from normality that rob the living organism of the unique property bestowed by this tissue is supremely rewarding. Science truly rejoins philosophy as our comprehension and appreciation of this remarkable tissue grow.

Although retinal biochemistry can now be considered as a speciality in its own right, this Symposium served to emphasize that even this relatively small field can be subdivided into several individual aspects, each with its own disciplines, techniques and literature. Such sub-fractionation is characteristic of the evolutionary pattern of all branches of science, and places even greater responsibility on the individual to communicate with his scientific neighbour. If science is synonymous with truth, it is essential that we learn to ask humbly and to give freely. That such an ideal can become reality was borne out by the sincerity and enthusiasm of all those who took part in this first Symposium. Any credit for the success of this venture, can, therefore, be shared equally between all those who participated.

The absence of a comprehensive basic literature on the biochemistry of the retina has frustrated the would-be disciple for many years. In view of the rapid recent expansion of the subject, the need for an adequate and concise literature has become increasingly imperative, and it was for this reason that this Symposium, in its present form, was first envisaged. It is hoped that from the 3 days in September in which this meeting took place, and now between the covers of this book, we have managed to collate both current and review aspects of the major topics of interest in retinal biochemistry. We have also included information from related fields from which we can no longer afford to isolate ourselves. It is intended that this Symposium should be the first of many that will provide future investigators, both in this and allied fields, with a continuous and informative literature, as well as a wealth of speculation that will provide the research worker with fuel for many years to come.

The meeting would not have been possible in the form it eventually took without the very generous assistance of Smith and Nephew Research Ltd. Although many people connected with this company assisted me, I would particularly like to thank Mr. E. M. Bavin and Mr. G. W. Billington for their invaluable liaison. It is never possible to thank all those concerned in a venture such as this, but I must acknowledge the tremendous encouragement of Professor Norman Ashton without whose continual support I would have lacked the presumption to continue with the task. Mr. Ralph Kissun, of my own laboratory, assisted in every phase of the operations, and I cannot overpraise his help and support. For help in a variety of ways, my thanks are due also to Miss Heather Brown, Mr. David Morley, Mr. Selwyn Henry and Mr. Walter Buchanan, as well as to many people in the "Institute" workshops who did not hesitate to provide "extra" assistance or advice when required.

My gratitude is due also to all those who participated in the discussions for allowing their comments to be recorded and possibly misinterpreted! The spontaneous comment rarely does justice to the speaker's beliefs, and if quoted out of context might well appear irrelevant or even uninformed. Although every effort has been made to record accurately the ideas of those who spoke, I must accept all responsibility for inadvertent misrepresentation, and ask for a degree of tolerance both on the part of the reader and the participant.

Lastly I would like to thank both Experimental Eye Research and Academic Press for their advice and co-operation in publishing these proceedings.

CLIVE N. GRAYMORE

List of Participants

Guest of Honour: PROFESSOR SIR CHARLES DODDS, M.V.O., F.R.S.

DR. A. AMES III, *Harvard Medical School, Boston, Mass., U.S.A.*

DR. G. ARDEN, *Institute of Ophthalmology, London, England*

PROFESSOR N. ASHTON, *Institute of Ophthalmology, London, England*

DR. R. BARRY, *Birmingham and Midland Eye Hospital, Birmingham, England*

DR. C. BRIDGES, *Institute of Ophthalmology, London, England*

MISS H. BROWN, *Institute of Ophthalmology, London, England*

PROFESSOR V. BONAVITA, *University of Palermo, Palermo, Italy*

DR. E. CAMERON, *Institute of Ophthalmology, London, England*

MISS E. BURDEN, *University College, London, England*

DR. D. CAMPBELL, *Birmingham and Midland Eye Hospital, Birmingham, England*

DR. C. CHLOUVERAKIS, *Guy's Hospital Medical School, London, England*

PROFESSOR L. COHEN, *University of Manitoba, Winnipeg, Man., Canada*

DR. D. COLE, *Institute of Ophthalmology, London, England*

DR. S. J. CREWS, *Birmingham and Midland Eye Hospital, Birmingham, England*

DR. CUNHA-VAZ, *Institute of Ophthalmology, London, England*

DR. A. G. EVERSON PEARSE, *Postgraduate Medical School, London, England*

MISS R. FIDDICK, *University College Hospital Medical School, London, England*

DR. S. FUTTERMAN, *Howe Laboratory of Ophthalmology, Boston, Mass., U.S.A.*

DR. C. N. GRAYMORE, *Institute of Ophthalmology, London, England*

MISS S. GUPTA, *University College, London, England*

DR. H. HEATH, *University College Hospital Medical School, London, England*

DR. P. HENKIND, *Institute of Ophthalmology, London, England*

DR. H. IKEDA, *Institute of Ophthalmology, London, England*

DR. H. KEEN, *Guy's Hospital Medical School, London, England*

DR. M. KERLY, *University College, London, England*

DR. T. KUWABARA, *Howe Laboratory of Ophthalmology, Boston, Mass., U.S.A.*

DR. Y. MANUEL, *France*

PROFESSOR H. McILWAIN, *Institute of Psychiatry, London, England*

DR. G. MORGAN, *Institute of Ophthalmology, London, England*

DR. N. MUKAI, *Institute of Ophthalmology, London, England*

PROFESSOR F. NEWELL, *University of Chicago, Chicago, Ill., U.S.A.*

DR. J. NEWHOUSE, *Royal College of Surgeons, London, England*

PROFESSOR W. K. NOELL, *State University of New York, Buffalo, N.Y., U.S.A.*

DR. FERRAZ DE OLIVEIRA, *Institute of Ophthalmology, London, England*

R. A. PATERSON, ESQ., *University College Hospital Medical School, London, England*

DR. C. PEDLER, *Institute of Ophthalmology, London, England*

PROFESSOR A. POTTS, *University of Chicago, Chicago, Ill., U.S.A.*

DR. H. READING, *Royal College of Surgeons, London, England*

DR. M. RILEY, *Institute of Ophthalmology, London, England*

A. RUTTER, ESQ., *University College Hospital Medical School, London, England*

DR. D. SEVEL, *Institute of Ophthalmology, London, England*

DR. MANOUCHER SHAKIB, *Institute of Ophthalmology, London, England*

A. SHEARER, ESQ., *Birmingham and Midland Eye Hospital, Birmingham, England*

DR. T. SLATER, *University College Hospital Medical School, London, England*

MISS E. TONKS, *Birmingham and Midland Eye Hospital, Birmingham, England*

DR. M. TOWLSON, *Institute of Ophthalmology, London, England*

PROFESSOR G. WALD, *Harvard University, Cambridge, Mass., U.S.A.*

Introductory Comments

Professor Norman Ashton

Director, Department of Pathology, Institute of Ophthalmology,
University of London, England

As a person mainly concerned with experimental pathology and morbid anatomy I cannot claim any special knowledge of recent advances in biochemistry, but I have two lame excuses for introducing this important meeting, the first international symposium on the biochemistry of the retina. To begin with, my colleague Dr. Graymore asked me to do so and it would be very difficult to refuse such a nice person, and secondly because for the last 15 years, that is just over 20% of threescore years and ten, I have been intensely interested in the normal and abnormal behaviour of the retina, much of which must eventually be explicable in terms of chemical events. In fact, it was the realization of the great need for more fundamental knowledge of the metabolism of the retina, a need highlighted by the discovery in 1953 that oxygen specifically affected its developing vessels, that led me exactly 8 years ago to seek the help of several distinguished scientists to find a young biochemist to devote himself fully to this particular tissue. That is how Dr. Graymore came to the Institute of Ophthalmology in London and into this field, and so in due course to originate and organize this first symposium.

It seems unbelievable now to recall how little was known at that time. Although the classic work of Warburg in 1924 had shown the uniquely high glycolytic and respiratory activity of this tissue, it was not until 1935 to 1940 that the operation of the normal Embden-Meyerhof sequence was established—Dr. Margaret Kerly's researches being prominent in achieving this—but the existence of an active Krebs cycle was not so readily confirmed owing to confusion in the differing behaviour of the retina *in vitro* in bicarbonate and phosphate buffers, as originally discovered by Laser. As recently as 1946, Krause and Sibley stated in a review that "oxidation probably does not take place through the Krebs' citric acid cycle", but it is now generally accepted that the reactivity in bicarbonate more nearly reflects normal metabolism, and that a highly active Krebs cycle does in fact function in the retina. By the end of the 1940's, therefore, the existence of the glycolytic and respiratory pathways was recognized, their very high activity acknowledged, and the characteristic Pasteur effect accepted, but our knowledge was still very rudimentary.

In the early years of the 1950's, Sir Hans Krebs, who some years previously had noted the exceptionally high content of glutamate in the retina, described with his co-workers its importance in relation to potassium and water balance, and about the same time Crane and Ball demonstrated the very high affinity of the retina for carbon dioxide. More recently these aspects have been further studied; some light has been shed on the possible significance of glutamate by Professors Cohen and Noell, and the bicarbonate effect has been extensively investigated by Dr. Kerly and her colleagues, and, incidentally, both these groups of workers have demonstrated the Crabtree effect in the retina.

More and more people have now become intrigued by this readily manipulated membrane and many new facts, related and unrelated, are pouring into the literature and gaining such momentum that this symposium, providing as it does a pause for reflection, an opportunity to ventilate ideas and to discuss controversial issues, has become quite essential.

There has been a most productive concentration upon the detailed analysis of individual reactions and of their associations with certain cells within the retina—what has been termed biochemical cytology—and particularly interesting comparative studies on pathological conditions of the retina have been reported. Dr. Lowry and his co-workers, for instance, have achieved a great deal, by the use of admirable micro-histological techniques, in localizing enzyme activity in particular layers (unfortunately he was not able to attend this meeting). Similar contributions of great value have been made, through the application of conventional histochemistry, by Dr. Kuwabara and his colleagues of Boston. He will be telling us of his work, and here we have the benefit of the presence of Dr. Everson Pearse, eminent exponent of this artistic science, and of Dr. Trevor Slater, who has worked for some years on the mechanisms of tetrazolium and related reactions.

Correlation of biochemical activity with morphological differentiation during development has been employed to advantage by Professor Cohen, Professor Noell, Dr. Graymore, and by Dr. Walters and Dr. Brotherton in Dr. Dorothy Campbell's unit at Birmingham, and they have furthered their studies by exploring the changes to be found in retinal degeneration, whether genetically controlled or chemically induced. Particularly interesting in this respect are the recent studies on hereditary degeneration in the rat, by Professor Bonavita, Dr. Reading and Dr. Graymore, wherein chemical changes have been shown to precede visible cell damage.

Several different chemical inhibitors have provided standard tools for examining the retina, and have been employed by many people here today, including Dr. Graymore, Dr. Newhouse, Dr. Potts (who will be mentioning his exciting studies in detail), and Professor Noell. The distinguished and well-documented work of Professor Noell on iodoacetate provides a classic example of the value of combining chemical, morphological and electro-physiological approaches in this field of study. Similar techniques have been used on the isolated retina by Dr. Ames, from whom we shall be hearing, while Dr. Arden and Dr. Ikeda will be talking about the use of electroretinograms and electrooculograms in the interpretation of retinal dystrophy. As shown by their interesting reports at Birmingham in 1964, Dr. Campbell and Miss Tonks have a foot in both the vitamin A and retinal dystrophy camps.

The activity of the alternative pathway, the pentose phosphate route, has been actively investigated in the last year or so by a number of workers here (Dr. Kerly, Dr. Futterman, Professor Noell, Professor Cohen, Dr. Graymore and Dr. Towlson). Dr. Futterman's work, relating the tissue metabolism to the visual cycle, is especially impressive, and we are fortunate to have Professor Wald and Dr. Bridges with us to keep an attentive ear on this part of the proceedings.

Coming more especially to the pressing problems of human disease—pressing because while we remain in ignorance in the laboratory little can be done for patients in the ward—we shall consider diabetic retinopathy, still one of the greatest challenges to medical science, and we look forward to the review of Dr. Keen, to the contributions of Dr. Heath and his collaborators from University College, and to hearing Professor Newell from Chicago who will be telling us more of his interesting work on glycogen synthesis in the retina.

Undoubtedly there is much to be learnt from biochemists working in other fields, for although different tissues have their specific metabolic features, they share common mechanisms, and much time might be saved by borrowing the experience of others, particularly from those concerned with the metabolism of the brain, of which the retina is but an extension. To ensure this extraretinal perception we hope that Sir Charles Dodds, Professor Wald and Professor McIlwain, will be joining us.

Here then at this small and informal symposium, the first of many to come, Dr. Graymore has prepared a menu to delight a glutton; and we hope the initiates and students present will find much to whet their appetites, for in the years ahead they in their turn will be organizing these symposia. Indeed it will give us the right atmosphere of humility to imagine how naive our deliberations today may then appear to them.

In looking to the future in this way, it would probably be right to guess that the electron microscope, with all its developing refinements, in obtaining yet higher and higher resolutions and in the elaboration of techniques for studying dynamic processes, will have much to contribute to our knowledge of the retina. The final unravelling of the maze of cellular interconnections alone must surely lead to new if not iconoclastic concepts of function, while the significance of many biochemical reactions cannot be properly understood without a knowledge of ultra-structure, as so clearly shown in the case of mitochondria and lysosomes. It is, therefore, a great pleasure for me to end this introduction by asking our own prospector in this relatively unexplored oil-field, Dr. Christopher Pedler, to open this meeting by telling us of his recent findings with the electron microscope.

Contents

Session 1. Chairman: Professor W. K. Noell

Session 2. Chairman: Dr. Dorothy Campbell

Session 3. Chairman: Dr. Margaret Kerly

Session 4. Chairman: Dr. S. Futterman

Session 5. Chairman: Dr. H. W. Reading

Rods and Cones—A Fresh Approach *

CHRISTOPHER PEDLER

Department of Anatomy, Institute of Ophthalmology, University of London, England

To explain duplex retinal properties it is assumed that there are two morphological varieties of receptor intimately associated with the phenomena of photopic and scotopic vision. The words 'rod' and 'cone', however, were first used by the light microscopist to describe nothing more than two cell varieties which could be distinguished by certain staining characteristics and the overall shape of part of the cell. Ever since, the terms, together with their implicit link with duplex retinal function and nocturnal and diurnal habit, have been adopted by workers from almost every discipline. The photochemist refers to *rod* and *cone* pigments without having any precise method of referring such pigments to a *particular* cell, at least until the advent of single-cell densitometry. The neurophysiologist, studying light-evoked retinal potentials, assumes the type of cell in the retina from which he has recorded his potentials, again without direct correlation between his findings and the actual receptors initiating the potential. Similarly, the electron microscopist describes fine structural distinctions between receptors, often dividing them again into two groups if at all possible. Thus, the rod and the cone have acquired a number of quite separate existences. They are morphological entities in the light and electron microscopes; they have a photochemical set of references; they are defined electrophysiologically; their presence or absence is predicted by animal behaviour and habit and their nature is assumed from the type of retina in which they are found.

There is, therefore, categorization without cross-reference showing an inbred bias towards the division of all phenomena into two classes to fit the concept of two receptor varieties. That photoreceptors cannot be completely divided into two classes is clear from the number of anomalies that exist among the vertebrate family.

The purpose of this article is to examine the internal components of some vertebrate photoreceptors as revealed by electron microscopy; to relate these to the concept of a 'rod' and 'cone'; and to consider some of the connections made by them in the outer plexiform layer.

Twenty-four species including man have been studied, and 9 major receptor components are considered.

Preliminary results from serial reconstruction of parts of 12 isolated Pigeon foveas are also reported, and the 'one-to-one' relationship of foveal receptors and bipolar processes is questioned on a cell-to-cell basis in this species.

By comparing these two groups of data with the anatomical relationships claimed by the light microscopist it is suggested that the concept of the 'rod' and 'cone' no longer fits the morphological facts well enough, and is due for replacement. It is also pointed out that some aspects of retinal cytology shown by the Golgi technique are, in the light of electron microscopic evidence, actively misleading and need to be modified.

---

* Abstract of lecture only. The content of the original lecture is reported in full elsewhere (Pedler, C., 1965. *Proceedings of the CIBA Symposium on the Physiology and Psychology of Vision.* In press.)

1

There are at least four varieties of process connecting with the surface of the synaptic pedicle: bipolar dendrites, horizontal cell processes, processes from the radial fibre complex and filaments from adjacent pedicles. There are, in addition, two morphological varieties of terminal at the pedicle surface. The filaments from adjacent pedicles are often recognizable since they also contain synaptic vesicles which are therefore found on both sides of the synaptic membranes. The processes from the horizontal cells are also frequently identifiable since they contain cytoplasmic constituents of a form unique to this region. The radial fibre processes can be often traced back to a main radial trunk, so we are left to account for the bipolar dendrites; these can end in either one of the two terminal varieties demonstrated. This abundance of connections is found only on the complex pedicles, and in the simple variety the type of terminal that inserts into the substance of the pedicle is the one most frequently found. However, it remains that allowing for the other three types of contact, bipolar contacts may number as many as 500. But we also know that bipolar domain overlap is considerable, even in central and para-foveal regions, and we have also seen that all the presumptively bipolar dendrites contacting a given pedicle originate from many bipolars, so that we have to conclude that a complex pedicle may, even in the fovea, release information to 30 or 40 bipolar cells at a conservative guess. Thus, assuming that a pedicle operates over its entire synaptic surface at once, the absorption of a spatially discrete spot of light in one receptor may activate literally hundreds of channels in the outer plexiform layer. The receptor with the complex pedicle therefore becomes a differentiator, and one with a simple pedicle, an integrator. But we have already encountered permutations of this general theme and must therefore complicate matters by speaking of three basic types which we have so far encountered, a sensitive multi-channel differentiator (type A), an insensitive multi-channel differentiator (type B) and a sensitive single-channel integrator (type C). The fourth logical variety, an insensitive single-channel integrator, will probably never be found, because there would be no need for summation under photopic conditions. One advantage of this scheme is that the many anomalies in the vertebrate family disappear because the cells are categorized by the electron microscopic features most surely related to function. We no longer have to force classical morphological duplicity on the sphenodon, the lung fish or the leopard frog, neither do we have to worry about such semantic absurdities as the rod-like cones of the primate and human foveae. It may be that the cell categories will have to be modified as more species are studied and as more is known about the photo-pigment content of individual outer segments and the nature of the information transfer at the synapses, but their use creates fewer anomalies than the concept of the rod and the cone which has served very well for nearly a century.

DISCUSSION

Dr. Arden opened the discussion by congratulating Dr. Pedler on advancing this most useful concept—it assisted one in understanding that the difference between photopic and scotopic vision should not be confined to the individuality of the receptors *per se*, but might also be a property of the neuronal interconnections. He added that the anomalies of structural interpretation to which Dr. Pedler had referred were also familiar in neurophysiology. In his own case, for example, he had been puzzled by the rod-like excitation and sensitivity of the Gecko cone. Dodt had also demonstrated cone-like responses in rod-like retinas. The elaborate cross-linkages revealed in the beautiful photographs of Dr. Pedler also served to explain why a single bipolar cell could be stimulated by light falling some distance away on the surface of the retina. Many points such

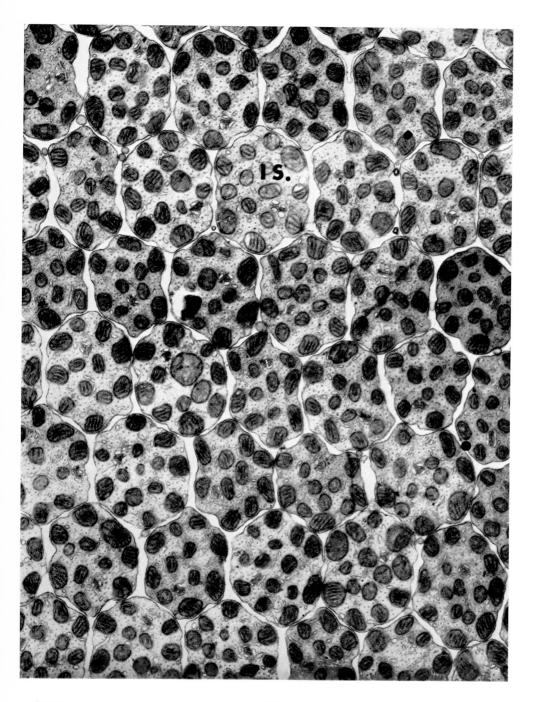

PLATE 1. A transverse section of inner segments (IS.), which are all of the same rod-like type, from a Bush baby (*Galago crassicaudatus agisymbanus* Coquerel). No large or cone-like varieties were found.

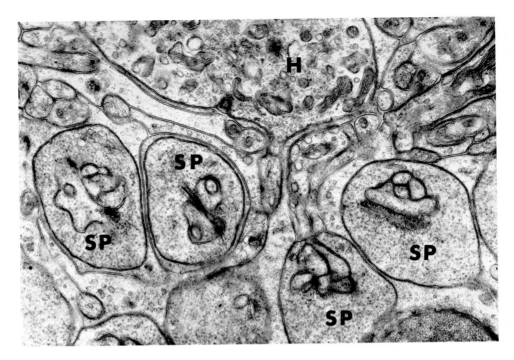

PLATE 2. Shows part of a horizontal cell (H) and several simple or rod-like receptor synapses (SP) which would be expected from the type of inner segment shown in Plate 1.

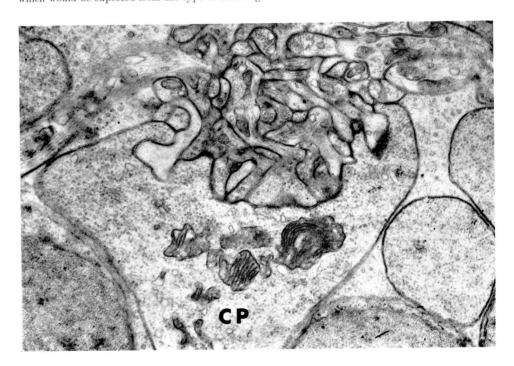

PLATE 3. Shows a complex or cone-like synaptic pedicle (CP) from the same tissue shown in Plates 1 and 2. One of these complex pedicles is found in approximately 40 simple pedicles. A finding that prevents the assumption that the Bush baby's receptors are all rods, and shows that receptors exist which are composite in type and can be called neither rod nor cone.

as these argued in favour of a very complex system of information-processing that was not revealed by earlier microscopic techniques, which tended to suggest an immediate association between receptor and nerve implying a one-to-one relationship.

PROFESSOR NOELL added that from the standpoint of the neurophysiologist one would never expect a simple one-to-one relationship between neurones. Excitatory and inhibitory impulses were required for any highly discriminatory process.

DR. HENKIND referred to Walls' idea of transformation of cones to rods, and queried the possibility that Dr. Pedler's third type of element might represent a transition form. He asked whether there was any evolutionary pattern indicating, for example, a smaller proportion of the third element in higher animals.

DR. PEDLER replied that he knew of no such pattern, and felt that Walls' theory was based on false premises and classification. Müller, he pointed out, had divided the receptors of the lamprey into rods and cones, and then reversed his decision some 5 years later. Dr. Pedler suggested that this uncertainty resulted from the fact that there was no real distinction. He believed that the morphological appearance in the lamprey merely represented a convenient stacking pattern for the curiously shaped receptors, reeulting in a staggering of elements designed to make the most use of available space. This gave the appearance of long and short members. It was this type of morphological inaccuracy which led to Walls' theory. He did not accept the transition idea in any way.

PROFESSOR NOELL pointed out that Dr. Pedler's classification was based on the synaptic region. Nevertheless one had to accept that one could distinguish between 'rods' and 'cones' by the light microscope, and also by the effect of inhibitors such as iodoacetate. He also wondered why, if one were considering transfer of information, Dr. Pedler had not used the very useful classification of Sjöstrand into α- and β-receptors. The α-receptors would represent Dr. Pedler's C-type and the β-receptors would include both A and B. He felt it should be stressed that no one feature could, or should, be used to provide an adequate classification.

DR. PEDLER explained that his intention was to avoid any one element, but rather to classify according to input, i.e., the outer segment, and the ultimate output *via* the synapse. Sjöstrand's classification was very ingenious, but nevertheless tended to ignore the outer segment and concern itself solely with classifying the synapse.

DR. BRIDGES added to the discussion by suggesting that a careful study of the visual pigments might be useful in classifying receptor cells. In response to a further question from DR. BRIDGES, DR. PEDLER said that his laboratory was in process of considering the pink and green rods of the frog from the standpoint of receptor pedicles. This was most interesting in view of the fact that this was an example of two different visual pigments occurring in the rod cell.

DR. KUWABARA questioned the classification of the incomplete lamellar elements as insensitive outer segments; he favoured the view that these were artefacts.

DR. PEDLER agreed that, at first, he too thought that these were artefacts, but that in view of the constancy of the picture obtained from well-preserved specimens of a truly duplex retina, having the pigment epithelium in place, one had to doubt the validity of this argument. Certainly, if they were artefacts, they were useful ones, reflecting some basic difference. It might be, he added, that the lamellar material was more sensitive to damage in the case of the cone outer segments. Nevertheless, this still represented a meaningful distinction.

PROFESSOR NOELL also asked about this point, and referred to some work by Japanese workers indicating that these invaginations might be related to the state of light or dark adaptation. DR. PEDLER said that his own studies had not revealed any such changes in the outer segments, although, he added, he had observed striking changes in the Müller fibres in light or dark adaptation. Although fibrils were apparent in the radial fibres of the lizard retina, for example, these became strikingly more apparent following 24 hr of dark adaptation—sufficiently different to enable the observer to determine the state of dark or light adaptation in these retinas.

PROFESSOR NOELL recalled that Lasansky and De Robertis had noted vesicle formation as an early change in animals treated with iodoacetate; Dowling had also observed this in hereditary degeneration in the rat.

DR. PEDLER thought this might be due to the condition of the tissue. He had noted that similar changes occurred after 7 days of culturing the retina, although he admitted that at this time considerable changes were evident elsewhere in the tissue.

Molecular and Kinetic Properties of NAD- and NADP-Linked Dehydrogenases in the Developing Retina*

Vincenzo Bonavita

Department of Neurology, University of Palermo, Palermo, Italy

Starch gel electrophoresis of LDH† and catalytic studies with purine and pyridine analogues of NAD have allowed a very early discrimination between normal rats and animals with inherited retinal degeneration, owing to the occurrence in the retina of dystrophic animals of a sharp shift of the isoenzymatic pattern toward the so-called "heart type".

In contrast with LDH, MDH has not revealed any consistent change of the per cent ratio between its components during the post-natal maturation of the normal and dystrophic retina. The same minor change of the enzyme affinity for oxaloacetate has been measured in both rat strains.

Determinations of the specific activities of MDH and GAPDH have not discriminated between normal rats and animals with inherited retinal degeneration. G6PDH and 6PDH have exhibited different developmental curves in the two strains. Normal animals have shown, in fact, the highest specific activity of both enzymes at birth, while rats with retinal dystrophy have attained the peak value of the two enzymes at the 12th day after birth with a subsequent decrease towards subnormal levels.

1. Introduction

Studies by Lowry, Roberts and Lewis (1956) and Lowry, Roberts, Schulz, Clow and Clark (1961) have emphasized that the chemical organization of the retina exhibits a compartmental arrangement with dramatic differences in the topographical distribution of enzymes.

In the present studies enzyme activities have been measured in the tissue as a whole, without considering the existence of metabolic compartments or pools. The use of macromethods does not permit detailed investigation of the various discrete layers of the retina. Such an experimental approach offers, however, valuable information especially in the neurochemical analysis of the inherited retinal degeneration of the rat; the present article is also concerned with this latter aspect.

Some of the observations described here have been reported previously (Bonavita, Ponte and Amore, 1963); other data refer to recent investigations of our laboratory, whose results are now in the press (Bonavita, Guarneri and Ponte, 1965).

2. Experimental

Experimental details concerning the source of chemicals, the technique of extraction of enzymes from retina, the conditions of starch gel electrophoresis of LDH and starch grain electrophoresis of MDH, the procedures for enzyme analysis and the method for nitrogen determinations have been published elsewhere (Bonavita et al., 1963; Bonavita Guarneri and Ponte, 1964, 1965).

* This investigation was aided by grants from the National Institute of Neurological Diseases and Blindness (grant B–2917) and the Consiglio Nazionale delle Ricerche (Roma).

† Abbreviations used: GAPDH, glyceraldehyde-3-phosphate dehydrogenase; G6PDH, glucose-6-phosphate dehydrogenase; LDH, lactate dehydrogenase; MDH, malate dehydrogenase; 6PDH, 6-phosphogluconate dehydrogenase, NAD, nicotinamide adenine dinucleotide; NADP, nicotinamide adenine dinucleotide phosphate.

3. Results

Lactate dehydrogenase

The results of quantitative determinations and electrophoretic and catalytic studies on LDH have been recently described elsewhere (Bonavita et al., 1963). A short summary is given here.

Measurements of total LDH specific activity do not clearly discriminate between normal animals and rats with inherited retinal degeneration until after the 22nd day of post-natal life. Electrophoretic and catalytic studies discriminate between the two strains much earlier. When LDH from the retina of adult rats is submitted to electrophoretic migration on starch gel at pH 8·6, under the experimental conditions noted above, four major peaks of enzyme activity are measured as separate components. A fifth fraction (isoenzyme 1) has been detected recently by cellulose acetate paper electrophoresis and direct visualization of enzyme activity on the supporting medium (Graymore, 1964). That this component, already shown in other central nervous tissues (Bonavita, Ponte and Amore, 1962), was truly lacking in the rat retina has been questioned previously by the author (Bonavita et al., 1963).

At birth, retinas from normal rats and animals with retinal dystrophy cannot be differentiated by their LDH patterns. This is not so, however, in a later stage of maturation. In fact, while the normal retina reveals a similar isoenzymatic pattern throughout development, LDH from the degenerating retina undergoes a quite early modification. Figure I illustrates the gradual evolution of the observed changes

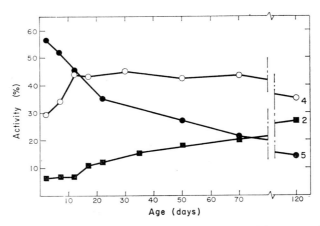

FIG. 1. Post-natal changes in the percentage activity of three LDH isoenzymes from the retina of rats with inherited retinal degeneration. Each experimental point represents the mean of at least three determinations on pools of 8–20 retinas (Bonavita, Ponte and Amore, 1963).

with the first appearance of a shift in the isoenzymatic composition before the tenth day of post-natal life. Similar data for retinal dystrophy have been reported also by Graymore (1964a, b).

Among the catalytic studies on LDH (Bonavita et al., 1963), the interaction with structural analogues of NAD seems to be particularly noteworthy. The reactivity of retina LDH with NAD analogues has shown definite differences between normal animals and rats with inherited retinal degeneration. Table I shows that the enzymes from new-born and mature retinas from normal animals have the same affinity for

NAD and other dinucleotides. It also shows that in the newborn LDH from the affected strain is identical with the enzyme of normal animals, while the reactivity of the enzyme from the mature degenerated tissue is substantially different.

TABLE I

Ratios of reaction rates measured with LDH from the retinas of new-born and adult rats after addition of 5 oxidized dinucleotides and two concentrations of L(+) lactate (Bonavita et al., 1963)

	$\dfrac{\text{NAD(L)}}{\text{NAD(H)}}$	$\dfrac{\text{APAD(L)}}{\text{APAD(H)}}$	$\dfrac{\text{Py3AlAD(L)}}{\text{Py3AlAD(H)}}$	$\dfrac{\text{TNAD(L)}}{\text{TNAD(H)}}$	$\dfrac{\text{NHD(L)}}{\text{NHD(H)}}$
Normal retina (2 days after birth)	0·38	1·23	0·20	0·20	0·25
Normal retina (adult rat)	0·39	1·24	0·20	0·20	0·28
Affected retina (2 days after birth)	0·38	1·23	0·20	0·19	0·24
Affected retina (adult rat)	0·61	1·30	0·26	0·24	0·47

The data collected in this table have been obtained by assaying the LDH activity with two concentrations of L(+) lactate (0·074 M and 0·0074 M, which are referred to as (H) and (L), respectively). All the data have been obtained in the presence of 0·7 μmoles of dinucleotide, and each value represents the mean of at least three determinations.

The abbreviations used for coenzyme analogues are: APAD, 3-acetylpyridine derivative; Py3AlAD, pyridine-3-aldehyde derivative; TNAD, thionicotinamide derivative; NHD, hypoxanthine derivative.

Glyceraldehyde-3-phosphate dehydrogenase, glucose-6-phosphate dehydrogenase and 6-phosphogluconate dehydrogenase

Though the significance of enzyme activities as measures of the capacity of metabolic pathways is highly questionable, another enzyme participating in glycolysis (GAPDH) and two enzymes operating in the "pentose phosphate pathway" (G6PDH and 6PDH) have been investigated.

Studies using [^{14}C]glucose have made it clear that the proportion of glucose metabolized through the pentose phosphate pathway is very small as compared to the glycolytic pathway (see Geiger, 1960). Findings of Hoskin (1960) and Cohen and Noell (1960) have strongly suggested, however, that the oxidative shunt, or part of it, may come into operation in the same nerve tissue under abnormal conditions. On these theoretical grounds, G6PDH and 6PDH in normal and degenerating retina appear worthy of consideration. Furthermore, interest in these two enzymes has been stimulated by the findings of Lowry et al. (1961) concerning the topographic distribution of G6PDH in the retina. The synapse between the visual cell and the bipolar cell is, in fact, surprisingly rich in the enzyme, thus suggesting that G6PDH and NADP may take part in the synaptic transmitter system (Noell, 1958).

GAPDH specific activity has exhibited the same developmental curve in normal and dystrophic retinas (Bonavita et al., 1965). G6PDH and 6PDH have shown, on the contrary, a consistent difference between normal and dystrophic rats. As shown in Figs. 2 and 3, a progressive drop of the two enzymes occurs in the normally developing retina whereas the specific activity of G6PDH and 6PDH increases in the degenerating retina until the 12th day of post-natal life and then falls to reach, by the 30th day, the values observed in normal animals.

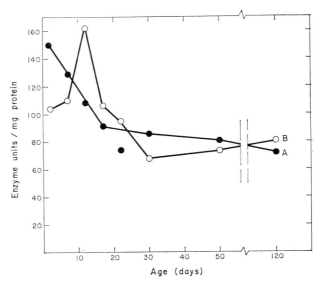

FIG. 2. Changes in G6PDH specific activity during the post-natal development of retina of normal and affected rats (A and B, respectively). Each experimental point represents the mean of two determinations on pools of 10–14 retinas. These measurements and the other enzyme determinations reported in this article have been performed at 25° (Bonavita et al., 1965).

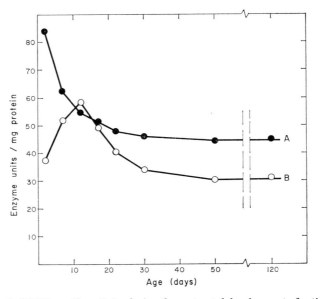

FIG. 3. Changes in 6PDH specific activity during the post-natal development of retina of normal and affected rats (A and B, respectively). For other details see Fig. 2 (Bonavita et al., 1965).

Malate dehydrogenase

Though existing in multiple forms, MDH can not be compared to lactate dehydrogenase. Electrophoretic species or isoenzymes of LDH appear, in fact, as gradually differentiated molecular types, while MDH exists in two main substantially different forms referred to as mitochondrial and supernatant enzymes (Englard, Siegel and Breiger, 1960; Grimm and Doherty, 1961; Delbrück, Schimassek, Bartsch and Bücher, 1959; Thorne, 1960; Johnson, 1962). Electrophoretic studies on starch grain have shown no differences between normal and dystrophic retinas. Figure 4

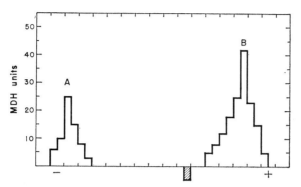

Fig. 4. Starch grain electrophoresis of MDH from retina of normal adult rats. The starting point is shown below the graph (Bonavita et al., 1965).

gives a diagrammatic representation of the electrophoretic pattern of the enzyme from the mature retina in the normal albino rat, but the same pattern has been found also with the mature dystrophic retina and the immature tissue of both rat strains. Similarly, the specific activity of MDH has shown no differences between the two strains. Malate dehydrogenation and oxaloacetate reduction have been measured at various developmental stages. As shown in Fig. 5, there is a significant elevation

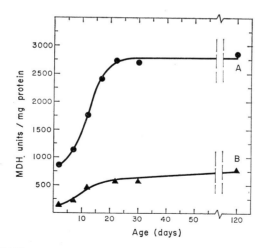

Fig. 5. Changes in MDH specific activity during the post-natal development of retina of normal rats. The upper curve refers to oxaloacetate reduction (●); the lower curve to malate dehydrogenation (▲) (Bonavita et al., 1965).

in activity with both substrates. There is, however, no difference between normal and dystrophic retinas. Figure 5 shows also that the ratio between oxaloacetate reduction and malate dehydrogenation decreases progressively. This decrease and the decrease of enzyme affinity for oxaloacetate are almost coincident (Bonavita et al., 1965).

4. Discussion

As mentioned previously, Graymore (1964a,b) has observed in the dystrophic retina electrophoretic changes of LDH similar to those described by Bonavita et al. (1963) and briefly summarized in the present report. Graymore (1964a,b) has found, however, through a direct visualization of enzyme activity on cellulose acetate paper, that also in normal rats LDH isoenzyme 5 (the so-called 'muscle type' enzyme) (Cahn, Kaplan, Levine and Zwilling, 1962) undergoes a smaller post-natal decrease which has not been noticed under our experimental conditions (see above). There is no easy explanation of such a disagreement.

Recent investigations in our laboratory have made it clear that the speed of LDH maturation is not the same in different nervous structures, the maturation of diencephalon being faster than that of other brain areas (Bonavita, Ponte and Amore, 1964). According to our findings, normal retina would appear, therefore, as the specialized portion of the central nervous system in which the molecular maturation of LDH is essentially pre-natal.

The physiological significance of electrophoretic and catalytic changes in the dystrophic retina as compared to normal retina has been discussed elsewhere (Bonavita et al., 1963) and will not be reconsidered in detail. Among the various findings the early occurrence of a drop of isoenzyme 5 in the degenerating retina seems particularly noteworthy. This decrease is measured even earlier than the decrease of anaerobic glycolysis (Walters, 1959; Graymore and Tansley, 1959; Graymore and Towlson, 1963; Brotherton, 1962), and before the first morphological signs of disease which have been observed in animals at the age of 12 days by the electron-microscope (Dowling and Sidman, 1962). Though we cannot establish the role of LDH *per se* in the inherited retinal degeneration, it is worth mentioning that an alteration of the electrophoretic pattern of the enzyme has been recently observed in other inherited diseases such as human muscle dystrophy (Wieme and Herpol, 1962) and hereditary muscle dystrophy of the chicken (Kaplan and Cahn, 1963).

The results concerning the other enzymes participating in glucose metabolism deserve a shorter comment. Measurements of GAPDH specific activity have not discriminated between normal and dystrophic retinas at any development stages after birth. It would seem, therefore, that the fall of anaerobic glycolysis observed by Walters (1959), Graymore and Tansley (1959) and Brotherton (1962) in the degenerating retina cannot be attributed to a selective decrease of this enzyme. Although any comparison between histochemical data and specific activity measurements is extremely arbitrary, it is worth mentioning in this connection that Forgsac (1963) has recently obtained histochemical evidence of a GAPDH fall in retinal degeneration induced by mono-iodoacetate.

G6PDH and 6PDH have shown almost the same developmental curve when measured in each of the two investigated strains. By contrast, a significant difference has been found between normal rats and animals with inherited retinal degeneration. In the dystrophic retina G6PDH reaches its peak value (the same value observed at birth in normal rats!) only at the 12th day of post-natal life, and then decreases toward the values measured in normal animals. The same behaviour is exhibited by 6PDH, although lower values are measured in the dystrophic retina at all developmental stages. Interestingly enough, the highest level of these two enzymes is measured in the dystrophic retina when lactate dehydrogenase of the muscle type is markedly decreasing. This could indicate a transitory substitutive role of the glucose oxidative shunt when the glycolytic capacity of the tissue decreases as shown by metabolic and enzymological studies (Brotherton, 1962; Bonavita et al., 1963; Graymore, 1964a,b).

The progressive post-natal decrease of G6PDH and 6PDH in the normal developing retina is also particularly noteworthy. It is in keeping with studies by Cohen and Noell (1960) and Graymore and Towlson (1963), who have shown that the alternative pathway of glucose breakdown plays a more significant role in the retina of the immature as compared to the adult animals.

In contrast with LDH, MDH has not shown developmental changes of its electrophoretic pattern nor has it discriminated between the normal and dystrophic tissue. Recent data from this laboratory have made it clear, in fact, that the situation of MDH is to be generally contrasted with that of LDH from the embryological viewpoint (Bonavita, Guarneri and Ponte, 1964). Moreover, it is not possible to discriminate between normal and dystrophic retinas even when catalytic features such as the affinity for malate and oxaloacetate have been measured, although a change does occur in the developing enzyme as shown by the increase of the Michaelis constant for oxaloacetate. That normal and dystrophic retinas cannot be distinguished by electrophoretic studies on MDH, however, loses part of the significance which one would attribute to it at first sight, when considering the relative stability of MDH patterns in other developing tissues (Bonavita, Guarneri and Ponte, 1964).

The present findings on MDH deserve a short comment also from a metabolic view-point. While electrophoretic patterns of the developing retina have not given any significant information as to whether the ratio between mitochondrial and cytoplasmic MDH is changing, the observed decrease of the affinity for oxaloacetate suggests the occurrence of an increase of the mitochondrial enzyme, which could also cause a change in the efficiency of the so-called "malate-oxaloacetate shuttle system" (Kaplan, 1961). It seems quite questionable, however, that this system is truly operating *in vivo*, since it requires each molecular species of MDH to be present in one cellular compartment, and this has not been proved to be so in a recent investigation on the brain enzyme (Bonavita, Guarneri and Ponte, 1964).

In conclusion, studies on MDH do not contribute to the analysis of the metabolic organization of the retina as do studies on other enzymes.

ACKNOWLEDGMENTS

The author wishes to acknowledge the collaboration of Dr. G. Amore, Dr. R. Guarneri and Dr. F. Ponte in different aspects of this work

REFERENCES

Bonavita, V., Guarneri, R. and Ponte, F. (1964). *Acta Embryol. Morph. exp.* **7**, 258.
Bonavita, V., Guarneri, R. and Ponte, F. (1965). *Vision Res.* **5**, 113.
Bonavita, V., Ponte, F. and Amore, G. (1962). *Nature, Lond.* **196**, 576.
Bonavita, V., Ponte, F. and Amore, G. (1963). *Vision Res.* **3**, 271.

Bonavita, V., Ponte, F. and Amore, G. (1964). *J. Neurochem.* **11**, 39.

Bourne, M. C., Campbell, D. A. and Tansley, K. (1938). *Br. J. Ophthal.* **23**, 613.

Brotherton, J. (1962). *Exp. Eye Res.* **1**, 246.

Cahn, R. D., Kaplan, N. O., Levine, L. and Zwilling, E. (1962). *Science* **136**, 962.

Cohen, L. H. and Noell, W. K. (1960). *J. Neurochem.* **5**, 253.

Delbrück, A., Schimassek, H., Bartsch, K. and Bücher, T. (1959). *Biochem. Z.* **331**, 297.

Dowling, J. E. and Sidman, R. L. (1962). *J. cell Biol.* **14**, 73.

Englard, S., Siegel, L. and Breiger, H. H. (1960). *Biochim. biophys. Acta* **56**, 571.

Forgacs, J. (1963) *Experientia* **19**, 236.

Graymore, C. N. and Tansley, K. (1959). *Br. J. Ophthal.* **43**, 177.

Graymore, C. N. and Towlson, M. (1963). *Exp. Eye Res.* **2**, 48.

Graymore, C. N. (1964a). *Nature, Lond.* **201**, 615.

Graymore, C. N. (1964b). *Exp. Eye Res.* **3**, 5.

Grimm, F. C. and Doherty, D. G. (1961). *J. biol. Chem.* **236**, 1980.

Hoskin, F. C. G. (1960). *Biochim. biophys. Acta* **40**, 309.

Johnson, M. K. (1962). *Biochem. J.* **84**, 25P.

Kaplan, N. O. (1961). In *Mechanism of Action of Steroid Hormones*, p. 247. Pergamon Press, Oxford.

Kaplan, N. O. and Cahn, R. D. (1962). *Proc. nat. Acad. Sci. U.S.A.* **48**, 2123.

Lowry, O. H., Roberts, R. N., and Lewis, C. (1956). *J. biol. Chem.* **220**, 879.

Lowry, O. H., Roberts, R. N., Schulz, D. W., Clow, J. E. and Clark, J. R. (1961). *J. biol. Chem.* **236**, 2813.

Noell, W. K. (1958). *Arch. Ophthal.* **60**, 702.

Thorne, C. J. R. (1960). *Biochim. biophys. Acta* **42**, 175.

Walters, P. T. (1959). *Br. J. Ophthal.* **43**, 686.

Wieme, R. J. and Herpol, J. E. (1962). *Nature, Lond.* **194**, 287.

DISCUSSION

DR. GRAYMORE said that the studies on the isoenzyme patterns of lactic dehydrogenase of the retina of normal and dystrophic rats carried out in his own laboratory agreed essentially with the findings of Professor Bonavita. The technique of electrophoresis on cellulose acetate paper that he had employed carried the advantages of speed and simplicity, although the accuracy of the assay, even after elution with alcohol, was probably below that obtained using more conventional techniques. He pointed out, however, that the choice of this technique demonstrated quite clearly the presence of a fraction 1, the 'heart isoenzyme'. This was apparent whether the strips were merely examined visually, or specrophotometrically following elution. A further difference concerned the developmental pattern of LDH 5 in both normal and dystrophic retinae. Although the activity of this fraction was always lower in retinas from retinitis animals than from normal animals, at all stages of development examined, the absolute level of activity fell progressively during development in both normal and dystrophic retinas. This, he thought, might be related to synthetic processes concerned in tissue differentiation.

Dr. Graymore added that malate dehydrogenase had also been studied in his laboratory, using the same technique of separation on cellulose acetate paper. Homogenization with either glass distilled water or isotonic saline had clearly defined the presence of both a soluble and a mitochondrial fraction and in agreement with Professor Bonavita there was no difference in pattern between retinal extracts from normal and dystrophic animals.

DR. FUTTERMAN suggested that, in view of the basic effect on the outer limbs in this condition, it might well be worthwhile investigating isoenzyme patterns in these elements. The observed overall effect might well reflect some more acute condition in the outer segments. PROFESSOR BONAVITA doubted the likelihood of such investigations being of value, however, on the grounds that the changes in isoenzyme patterns reported preceded by several days the observed morphological changes.

DR. ARDEN challenged Professor Bonavita's objection, pointing out that electrophysiological determinations suggested that there may be some biochemical defect long before structural changes became apparent. On the grounds that this retinal dystrophy might well result from a primary disturbance of the pigment epithelium, for example, he felt that investigations of this particular layer might well be of value. He agreed, however, that there were considerable difficulties both as regards separation technique and the quantity of tissue available.

DR. FUTTERMAN, in reply to a question from PROFESSOR NOELL regarding the purity of the outer segment preparations, assured the meeting that providing the homogenate was prepared in isotonic medium, the outer segments appeared to retain considerable activity. Hypotonic solutions could then be employed to leach out the water-soluble enzymes required for study. He felt that about 10 rat retinas would be required for these determinations.

DR. READING thought that although changes in the pattern of isoenzyme distribution had occurred at an early stage, was it not true that overall lactic acid production was a more reliable parameter of retinal function, and reminded the meeting that this facet had not been shown to alter until a late stage in the lesion. Dr. Reading felt that systems more directly coupled metabolically with the shunt mechanism would prove ultimately to be of greater importance. In muscular dystrophy, for example, although a change in isoenzyme pattern was known to occur, the primary error appeared to lie in a leakage of creatine kinase. In this sense, he felt that the isoenzyme change in retinal dystrophy would prove to be secondary, and that some other mechanisms intimately connected with the shunt mechanism would be primary. PROFESSOR BONAVITA explained that he agreed with such criticism, but stressed that he was merely reporting the earliest changes so far detected in this disease. It was quite possible that even earlier aberrations would be noted, that may well assist an understanding of the aetiology of the condition, but meanwhile such observations as those reported were of value.

PROFESSOR COHEN asked Dr. Futterman, in relation to his comment on analysis of outer segment preparations, what his views were concerning the significance of contamination of such preparations by inner segment material. He felt that the high activity of the latter might represent a real hazard in such studies, as Dr. Futterman had pointed out in one of his papers. DR. FUTTERMAN agreed that it was difficult to ignore the possibility of contamination, but that in those systems he had examined, isolation and repeated washing in isotonic media indicated that a certain level of activity remained. On the basis of a simple interpretation this would suggest that intrinsic qualities were revealed.

PROFESSOR COHEN asked whether hexokinase or phosphofructokinase had been studied in the developing retina. Both these enzymes had been implicated in regulatory mechanisms, and in the former case the enzyme had been shown to be of importance in inducing other substrate levels which in turn would become rate-limiting. Both PROFESSOR BONAVITA and DR. KERLY said they were studying these systems in the dystrophic retina.

DR. TOWLSON closed the discussion, and suggested that in view of the selective destruction of the rod cells in retinitis pigmentosa, would it not be of interest to study isoenzyme patterns in pure rod and pure cone retinas?

The Activity of NADH-Monodehydroascorbic Acid-Transhydrogenase in Retinal and Ciliary Microsomes*

H. HEATH AND R. FIDDICK

*Department of Chemical Pathology, University College Hospital Medical School,
London, England*

Ascorbic acid is known to occur in high concentrations in ocular tissues but the function which this vitamin plays in ocular metabolism has not as yet been elucidated. In recent years, ascorbic acid-dependent NADH oxidizing systems have been demonstrated in animal (Staudinger, Krisch and Leonhäuser, 1961) and plant (Nason, Wosilait and Terrell, 1954; Kern and Racker, 1954) tissues. Staudinger et al. (1961) have shown that adrenal microsomes are only able to oxidize NADH in the presence of ascorbic acid. Since this reaction is not inhibited by cyanide, and dehydroascorbic acid does not act as the electron acceptor, these workers have been able to demonstrate that ascorbic acid is oxidized by the cyanide-insensitive, autoxidizable cytochrome b_5 to the free radical, monodehydroascorbic acid, which is subsequently reduced by NADH-monodehydroascorbic acid-transhydrogenase. The net result is that the ascorbic acid takes part in a cyanide-insensitive, reversible oxidation and reduction, with the concomitant oxidation of the pyridine nucleotide and the reduction of the cytochrome. The oxygen consumption of the retina, ciliary processes, cornea and lens is not completely inhibited by cyanide and it was therefore decided to investigate the possible presence of a cyanide-insensitive, ascorbic acid-dependent NADH oxidizing system in ocular tissues.

NADH-monodehydroascorbic acid-transhydrogenase has been shown to be present in the microsomal fraction from ocular tissue homogenates, and was most active in the preparations from the retina and ciliary processes. NADPH could not replace NADH, and cysteine, reduced glutathione, ergothioneine and dehydroascorbic acid could not be substituted for ascorbic acid in the reaction. The presence of cytochrome b_5 in retinal microsomes has been established. NADH-monodehydroascorbic acid-transhydrogenase was not inhibited by 0·1 M urethane, 10 mM malonate, 1·0 mM amytal, cyanide, cortisone, cortisol, 11-deoxycorticosterone and dexamethasone, but 0·1 mM p-chloromercuribenzoate and 1·0 mM iodoacetate exerted 81 and 33% inhibition, respectively, on the reaction. This enzyme system was also partially inhibited by low concentrations of Diamox and by high concentrations of chloroquine.

Full details of the experimental procedures and of the results obtained have been presented elsewhere and the possible role of this enzyme in secretory mechanisms has been discussed (Heath and Fiddick, 1964, 1965).

REFERENCES

Heath, H. and Fiddick, R. (1964). *Nature, Lond.* **202**, 1128.
Heath, H. and Fiddick, R. (1965). *Biochem. J.* **94**, 114.
Kern, M. and Racker, E. (1954). *Arch. Biochem. Biophys.* **48**, 235.
Nason, A., Wosilait, W. D. and Terrell, A. J. (1954). *Arch. Biochem. Biophys.* **48**, 233.
Staudinger, H., Krisch, K. and Leonhäuser, S. (1961). *Ann. N. Y. Acad. Sci.* **92**, 195.

*This work was supported by grants from the Medical Research Council and the British Foundation for Research into the Prevention of Blindness.

DISCUSSION

DR. RILEY referred to work by de Roetth on the ox retina and said that he had decided to have another look at the cyanide insensitive respiration of the ciliary processes. He had confirmed de Roetth's work obtaining an 82% inhibition of respiration in the whole tissue incubated in the presence of cyanide. He found, however, that Diamox did not significantly increase this inhibition in such whole tissue preparations, although he thought it would be of interest to repeat these experiments in the presence of ascorbate and NADH.

PROFESSOR NEWELL explained that work in his own laboratory tended to suggest that chloroquine exerted its effect at the level of synthetic processes rather than energy yielding mechanisms. Although chloroquine reached a level of 10^{-3} M or more in the pigmented structures, the dissociation constant was quite small, and he felt the effect was probably secondary due to the release of small quantities over a long period of time, rather than a result of the high concentrations used in enzyme studies.

Stoichiometry of Retinal Vitamin A Metabolism during Light-adaptation*

Sidney Futterman

Howe Laboratory of Ophthalmology, Massachusetts Eye and Ear Infirmary and Harvard Medical School, Boston, Mass., U.S.A.

The equilibrium constant for the alcohol dehydrogenase reaction at pH 7·4 is approximately 1. However, the ratio of free vitamin A to vitamin A aldehyde present at physiological pH in the light-adapted retina is greater than that predicted from the equilibrium of the alcohol dehydrogenase reaction. Vitamin A aldehyde, vitamin A, and vitamin A esters are not similarly distributed in the light-adapted retina. The results are in accord with the concept that vitamin A formed from vitamin A aldehyde in the outer segments of the visual cells must leave that compartment during light-adaptation and enter the microsomes where vitamin A ester is synthesized.

1. Introduction

The principal pathway of vitamin A metabolism in the retina which occurs during light-adaptation can be depicted as follows:

$$\text{Rhodopsin} \xrightarrow{\text{light}} \text{opsin} + \text{vitamin A aldehyde} \xrightarrow{\text{TPNH}} \text{vitamin A}$$

$$\downarrow$$

$$\text{vitamin A esters.}$$

The second reaction, the enzymatic reduction of vitamin A aldehyde to vitamin A, is catalyzed by alcohol dehydrogenase (Bliss, 1951) and is reversible. The equilibrium of this reaction has been thought to lie far in the direction of vitamin A formation at physiological pH (Wald, 1960). In view of the fact that the principal reducing agent for vitamin A aldehyde in the visual cycle is now known to be TPNH rather than DPNH (Futterman, 1963), it seemed desirable to re-examine the reaction and to determine the equilibrium constant for the retinal alcohol dehydrogenase reaction with both DPNH and TPNH serving as reducing agents for vitamin A aldehyde. Based on this information and estimations of the quantities of vitamin A aldehyde, vitamin A, and vitamin A esters present in dark- and light-adapted retinal tissue, an attempt was made to explain the stoichiometry observed in retinal vitamin A metabolism.

2. Materials and Methods

Materials

Pyridine nucleotides were obtained from Sigma Chemical Co. All-*trans* vitamin A

* This study has been supported by United States Public Health Service grant N B-02769.

aldehyde and all-*trans* vitamin A were purchased from Distillation Products Industries. Liver alcohol dehydrogenase was a product of the Worthington Biochemical Corporation.

Methods

Retinal alcohol dehydrogenase. Calf retinal visual cell outer segments were prepared as described previously (Futterman, 1963), by using isotonic KCl instead of 0·25 M sucrose. A crude preparation of alcohol dehydrogenase was prepared by homogenizing the visual cell outer segments obtained from 50 eyes in 30 ml of water, centrifuging at 800 × **g** for 5 min to remove a small amount of debris, and then centrifuging at 80,000 × **g** for 15 min to recover an insoluble lipoprotein residue containing both the alcohol dehydrogenase activity and rhodopsin of the retina. This red residue was carefully scraped from a small layer of black pigment granules and was suspended in isotonic phosphate buffer of pH 7.4.

Liver and retinal alcohol dehydrogenase reaction mixtures. Reaction mixtures containing 1 μmole of either vitamin A aldehyde or vitamin A (10 μmoles/ml in 50% dioxane containing 2·5% Triton X-100), 1 or 10 μmoles of DPNH, DPN, or TPNH, either 1 mg of liver alcohol dehydrogenase or 12·6 mg of crude visual cell alcohol dehydrogenase, and isotonic phosphate buffer of pH 7·4 in a final vol of 3·0 ml were incubated at 37° with shaking until equilibrium was approached (180 min). The vitamin A aldehyde content of reaction mixtures was determined at suitable intervals by extracting 0·2 ml samples with 4·8 ml of *n*-propanol, centrifuging, and assaying the supernatant fluid with thiobarbituric acid (see Futterman and Saslaw, 1961).

Incubation of retinal tissue. Whole or homogenized dark-adapted calf retinas were incubated in 0·5 ml of isotonic Tris-Cl buffer of pH 7·4 for 90 min at 37° either in opaque containers or exposed to light (approximately 15 in below a 100-watt incandescent bulb).

Retinal tissue fractions. Retinal tissue from 8 eyes, after incubation as above, was homogenized in 15 ml of isotonic Tris-Cl buffer of pH 7·4. Nuclei and visual cell outer segments were sedimented together by centrifugation at 1600 × **g** for 10 min and separated from the supernatant fluid which contained the mitochondria and microsomes (Futterman, 1963). The nuclei + outer segment fraction was washed by homogenizing in 10 ml of buffer and recovered by centrifugation at 6000 × **g** for 5 min. The supernatant fluid fractions were combined.

Analysis of incubated retinas or retinal tissue fractions. Retinal tissue or tissue fractions were extracted with isopropanol and petroleum ether, a portion of the extract was subjected to alumina chromatography, and the vitamin A and vitamin A ester fractions were analyzed fluorimetrically (Futterman and Andrews, 1964). Retinal tissue or tissue fractions from duplicate reaction mixtures were extracted with *n*-propanol and analyzed for vitamin A aldehyde with thiobarbituric acid (Futterman and Saslaw, 1961). However, in the case of the retinal tissue fraction containing mitochondria, microsomes, and supernatant fluid, a portion of the extract was concentrated to dryness under a stream of nitrogen, dissolved in 3 ml of *n*-propanol, and then analyzed for vitamin A aldehyde.

3. Results

Alcohol dehydrogenase equilibrium

When equal quantities of vitamin A aldehyde and reduced pyridine nucleotides were incubated together in the presence of either liver or retinal alcohol dehydrogenase until equilibrium was approached (Table I), approximately half of the aldehyde was converted to vitamin A. When the reaction was studied in either direction and when either TPNH or DPNH was employed the equilibrium constant for the reaction was approximately 1. It was apparent that at physiological pH the equilibrium of the alcohol dehydrogenase reaction did not lie in the direction of vitamin A formation.

B

TABLE I

Equilibrium constant of the alcohol dehydrogenase reaction at pH 7·4

| Source of enzyme | Reactants | | | Relative concentration of aldehyde at equilibrium* | Equilibrium constant† |
	A	B	A/B		K
Liver	DPNH	+ Ald.	1	52	0.9
Liver	DPNH	+ Ald.	10	9	1.0
Liver	DPN	+ Vit. A	1	53	0.8
Visual cell	DPNH	+ Ald.	1	50	1.0
Visual cell	TPNH	+ Ald.	1	49	1.1

* % of total vitamin in form of aldehyde at equilibrium

$$\dagger \; K = \frac{(DPN) \quad (Vitamin\ A)}{(DPNH) \quad (Vitamin\ A\ aldehyde)}$$

Stoichiometry in the retina

In the intact dark-adapted calf retina (Table II) most of the vitamin A is present as vitamin A aldehyde in the form of rhodopsin. There are also small amounts of vitamin A and vitamin A esters. When dark-adapted calf retinal tissue is incubated in the light most of the aldehyde liberated from the bleached visual pigment is reduced to vitamin A. Although a considerable fraction of the vitamin A was converted to vitamin A ester the ratio of free vitamin A to vitamin A aldehyde, 3·4 in the light-adapted retina, was much higher than the ratio of 1 which had been anticipated from the study of the alcohol dehydrogenase reaction. It seemed possible that the pH in the tissue might be somewhat below that of the surrounding buffer. Under these conditions the equilibrium of the alcohol dehydrogenase reaction would lie in the direction of vitamin A formation. However, the ratio of vitamin A to vitamin A aldehyde was essentially the same when a homogenate of retinal tissue was incubated under the same conditions (Table II).

TABLE II

Concentration of vitamin A metabolites in incubated calf retinas

Conditions	Recovery of vitamin A, all forms mμ moles	Vitamin A aldehyde mole (%)	Vitamin A mole (%)	Vitamin A esters mole (%)
Incubated in dark	23	93	5	2
Incubated in light	21	15	54	31
Homogenate incubated in light	23	12	47	41

Distribution in the retina

One possible explanation for the high concentration of free vitamin A in the light-adapted retina was that the aldehyde might be localized in the visual cell outer segments where it is formed and where the alcohol dehydrogenase is localized (Futterman and Saslaw, 1961), whereas the vitamin A might diffuse out of the outer segments and be present in other compartments within the retina. To examine this idea, incubated retinal tissue was homogenized and separated by centrifugation into two fractions. The vitamin A aldehyde, as expected, was largely confined to the fraction containing the visual cell outer segments (Table III). The small quantity of aldehyde present in the mitochondria + microsomes + supernatant fluid fraction was probably the result of contamination of this fraction with fragmented outer segments that failed to sediment at 1600 × **g**. Vitamin A, although occurring in both fractions of light-adapted retinal tissue, was present in the outer segment-containing fraction in much higher concentration than vitamin A aldehyde. Vitamin A ester was found largely in the fraction containing the microsomes.

TABLE III

Distribution of vitamin A aldehyde, vitamin A, and vitamin A esters between outer segment and microsome + supernatant fluid-containing fractions from incubated calf retinas

Fraction	Metabolite*	Dark-adapted retina mole (%)	Light-adapted retina mole (%)
Nuclei + outer segments	Vit. A ald.	76†	9
	Vit. A	7	40
	Vit. A esters	4	7
Microsomes + mitochondria + supernatant fluid	Vit. A ald.	5	3
	Vit. A	3	14
	Vit. A esters	5	27

* Recoveries of vitamin A, all forms, were 20 mμ moles/retina from the dark-adapted tissue and 23 mμ moles/retina from the light-adapted tissue.

† Present largely as rhodopsin.

4. Discussion

In an earlier study (Bliss, 1951) in which the alcohol dehydrogenase reaction was studied in only one direction, the equilibrium seemed to lie in the direction of vitamin A. Most probably the substrate, vitamin A, was contaminated with degradation products which were enzymatically inactive but assayed as vitamin A with $SbCl_3$. The presence of degradation products with the same fluorescence as vitamin A in stored preparations of the vitamin has been described (Futterman, 1962). In the present study the reaction was studied in both directions. When vitamin A was employed as a substrate, it was withdrawn from a freshly opened ampule and appeared to be homogenous when examined by paper chromatography (Futterman, 1962). When the alcohol dehydrogenase reaction was permitted to approach equilibrium from either direction at pH 7·4 in the presence of either vitamin A aldehyde or vitamin A and an equal quantity of appropriate pyridine nucleotide, essentially equal quantities of vitamin A aldehyde and vitamin A were present at equilibrium. The similar results obtained with TPNH and DPNH were in accord with observations establishing that the standard potentials for the TPN $\rightleftarrows$ TPNH and DPN $\rightleftarrows$ DPNH half reactions are almost identical (Rodkey, 1959).

In the retina, as elsewhere, the DPN is predominantly in the oxidized form while the TPN is largely in the reduced form (Slater, Heath, and Graymore, 1962). If the relative concentrations of the pyridine nucleotides were essentially the same in the visual cell outer segments as reported for the retina as a whole, and represented equilibrium concentrations, the ratio of reduced to oxidized pyridine nucleotide should be 0·3. Accordingly, the expected ratio of vitamin A to vitamin A aldehyde in the outer segments might be approximately 0·3. The observed ratio of vitamin A to vitamin A aldehyde was approximately 4. From this observation one might suspect either that the relative concentrations of the pyridine nucleotides differ considerably in the visual cell outer segments from those reported for the whole retina or that the alcohol dehydrogenase equilibrium is governed primarily by the TPNH, TPN system. The ratio of TPNH to TPN in rat retinal tissue (Slater et al., 1962) is approximately 3 and would be in accord with a vitamin A to vitamin A aldehyde ratio of the same magnitude.

In any case it is now clear that vitamin A aldehyde, vitamin A, and vitamin A ester are not similarly distributed in the retina. Vitamin A aldehyde is localized in the visual cell outer segments where the visual pigment and alcohol dehydrogenase reaction occur. The site of vitamin A esterification is now known to be in the microsomes (Andrews and Futterman, 1964). Vitamin A, therefore, must traverse the distance between these organelles. It is not surprising that vitamin A appears to be more widely distributed in the retina than is the aldehyde. Vitamin A ester appears to be present in the fraction containing microsomes. To account for these observations the existing concept of the visual cycle must be enlarged to include the interaction of at least two compartments within the retina (Fig. 1).

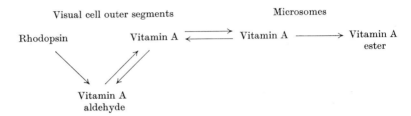

Fig. 1. Compartmentalized representation of retinal vitamin A metabolism in the visual cycle during light-adaptation.

REFERENCES

Andrews, J. S. and Futterman, S. (1964). *Fedn Proc. Fedn Am. Socs exp. Biol.* **23**, 527.
Bliss, A. F. (1951). *Arch. Biochem.* **31**, 197.
Futterman, S. (1962). *J. biol. Chem.* **237**, 677.
Futterman, S. (1963). *J. biol. Chem.* **238**, 1145.
Futterman, S. and Andrews, J. S. (1964). *J. biol. Chem.* **239**, 81.
Futterman, S. and Saslaw, L. D. (1961). *J. biol. Chem.* **236**, 1652.
Rodkey, F. L. (1959). *J. biol. Chem.* **234**, 677.
Slater, T. F., Heath, H. and Graymore, C. N. (1962). *Biochem. J.* **84**, 37P.
Wald, G. (1960). *Vitams Horm.*, **18**, 417.

DISCUSSION

In answer to a query from Professor Potts, Dr. Futterman assured the meeting that the pigment epithelium was not required for the synthesis of vitamin A ester. Krinsky had looked for a hydrolysing enzyme for the ester in pigment epithelium and not found one and it seemed unlikely that there was a hydrolysis and resynthesis in the pigment layer. He admitted, however, that it was difficult to assess the role of the pigment epithelium in the whole process. It would seem that it was required for removing vitamin A from the β-lipoprotein of the blood, and that esterification was probably a pre-requisite for migration into the retina. In answer to a further question from Professor Potts regarding the transport of free vitamin A, Dr. Futterman said he did not feel there was yet any convincing evidence of such a transference between the retina and pigment epithelium. The pigment epithelium appeared to contain only the esterified form, and certainly contained a very potent esterifying system. In light-adaptation, it was the ester that collected in the pigment layer, and there was no evidence for hydrolysis or resynthesis in that zone. In answer to a further question from PROFESSOR NOELL regarding Dowling's work on vitamin A diffusion, DR. FUTTERMAN agreed that this careful work suggested migration, but that these experiments had been carried out on the rat. No similar work had been done on other species.

DR. ARDEN questioned the value of the equilibrium constants quoted by Dr. Futterman, on the grounds that the *in vivo* compartmentation would invalidate any conclusions based on such figures. DR. FUTTERMAN agreed with this criticism and clarified the means by which the aldehyde might be removed from the original reaction.

DR. READING asked about the precise localization of the isomerization and its exact position in the sequence of events. DR. FUTTERMAN explained that the isomerization is thought to occur in the aldehyde stage and that in cattle this was known to occur in the retina.

DR. BRIDGES emphasized the inability of isolated outer limbs to regenerate visual purple—the pigment epithelium was essential and had been shown in the frog to contain the retinene isomerase. This enzyme is specific for retinene. It seemed unlikely, he added, that the vitamin A removed to the pigment layer would then be re-converted to retinene prior to isomerization, then converted back to the alcohol and esterified for transfer to the retina. This seemed a very complicated picture of little intrinsic value.

PROFESSOR COHEN thought that in view of the obvious reactivity of the aldehyde, one might speculate that reduction to the alcohol or the acetate was a prerequisite for transport.

DR. ARDEN suggested that one was making the system over complex by invoking this degree of compartmentation. He stressed the intimate contact of the pigment epithelium and outer limbs, and suggested that this relationship might well hold the key to the whole transformations.

Studies of Morphology, Chemistry and Function in Isolated Retina*

Adelbert Ames, III

Department of Biological Chemistry, Harvard Medical School, and Neurosurgical Service, Massachusetts General Hospital, Boston, Mass., U.S.A.

Methods are described for isolating rabbit retina and maintaining it for several hours *in vitro*. Two types of chambers have been used for recording light-evoked electrical responses either from the retina or from the attached segment of optic nerve. On the basis of morphological, chemical and electrical criteria, it appears possible to maintain the isolated retina in a condition closely approximating to its normal physiological state.

Three studies are briefly cited to indicate possible applications of this preparation. (1) Movements of water and electrolytes across retinal cell membranes were measured in response to an induced change in medium osmolality. (2) Changes in the light-evoked electrical response, during and after O_2 and/or glucose deprivation, were measured. (3) Changes in electron microscopic appearance associated with temporary deprivation of O_2 and glucose were examined.

1. Introduction

Among its many distinguishing features, the retina offers a peculiar practical advantage as an experimental preparation. It is probably the best suited of all organized mammalian tissues for study *in vitro*. It is remarkably thin and in some species has virtually no penetrating vessels but is nurtured, even *in vivo*, by diffusion from vascular networks on either surface. It can be separated from adjacent tissues without much trauma, and replacement of nutrition by diffusion, as it occurs *in vivo*, with nutrition by diffusion from a medium appears to be a relatively benign change.

In vitro study offers several distinct advantages if the tissue under examination can be maintained in a reasonably physiological state: (1) the chemical and physical milieu can be precisely defined and a single quantified experimental variable introduced; (2) certain metabolic and functional parameters can be monitored continuously during incubation (e.g., O_2 consumption, isotope exchange, electrical response); (3) analytically useful substances, such as an extracellular marker, a labeled substrate, or an histological fixative, can easily be introduced; (4) the tissue can be removed atraumatically at any instant in the course of the experiment for chemical or morphological examination.

Methods developed for isolating and incubating rabbit retina will be described and 3 studies exemplifying ways in which this preparation has been used will be reported briefly.

2. Methods

Rabbits were selected because they are readily available and have large retinas. The choice of this species has also enabled us to profit from the considerable volume of published information on rabbit retina, particularly the work from Dr. Werner K. Noell's laboratory. (e.g. Cohen and Noell, 1960; Noell, this Symposium.)

* These studies were supported in part by research grants (M-6209, MH-K3-3769) from the National Institute of Mental Health.

Under anesthesia, the conjunctiva is reflected and the major extraocular muscles are ligated and cut. The eye is then rapidly enucleated and placed in the combination slicer and dissection cup shown in Fig. 1. This provides for reproducible sectioning of the globe

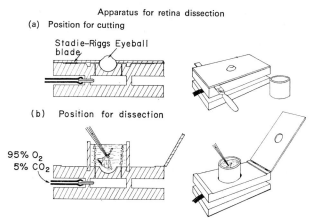

Apparatus for retina dissection

(a) Position for cutting

Stadie–Riggs Eyeball blade

(b) Position for dissection

95% O_2
5% CO_2

Fig. 1. Apparatus used first for hemisecting globe and then as a dissection dish for separating retina and attached segment of optic nerve from surrounding tissues.

without deformation. The front half of the eye is discarded, and the vitreous is removed *en masse* from the posterior half which has been maintained in its original hemispheric shape. The slicer is then immediately converted into a dissection cup and filled with medium which is kept equilibrated with an appropriate gas phase as shown. Under medium, the posterior half of the eye is everted over the rounded end of a Teflon rod, and that portion of the retina which has not separated spontaneously from the pigment epithelium and choroid is gently teased away with a smooth glass rod. The choroid and sclera are cut from the preparation at the disc. The segment of optic nerve is left attached to be used as a handle and for electrical recording, but is cut off before the tissue is subjected to chemical analysis. When isolating the retina under dim red light to preserve dark adaptation, it is helpful to illuminate the transparent dissection cup from below and to perform much of the dissection in silhouette. It is possible to isolate retinas from dark adapted rabbits and to incubate them for several hours in the dark while preserving a high rhodopsin content as indicated by their deep red color and low threshold of stimulation.

The composition of the medium is shown in the Table. It is maintained in equilibrium with a gas phase of 5% CO_2 and 95% O_2. Though a mixture of 5% CO_2 in air preserved

TABLE

Composition of medium

	Na^+	143·0	Cl^-	125·4
mequiv./1. of	K^+	3·6	HCO_3^-	22·6
solution	Ca^{++}	2·3	$H_2PO_4^-$	0·1
	Mg^{++}	2·4	$HPO_4^=$	0·8
			$SO_4^=$	2·4
	Total	151·3		151·3
mosmole/1. of	Electrolytes		298·7	
solution	Glucose		10·0	
		Total	308·7	

normal water and electrolyte distributions and the light-evoked electrical response recorded directly from the retina, the higher O_2 tension was found necessary for good preservation of the light-evoked response in the nerve.

Unusual precautions to eliminate toxic contaminants were found to be necessary for
these studies, and many of the procedures have been adapted from those used in tissue
culture work. The medium is carefully prepared with biological grade reagents and glass
redistilled water, and it comes in contact only with materials that have been proven to be
non-toxic and that have been carefully washed and rinsed. For example, the use of Ag,
AgCl electrodes is avoided since they cause rapid deterioration of the electrical response.

Just before introducing the medium, the entire incubating set-up is rinsed with fresh
human plasma. This was found necessary for the maintenance of a normal electrical
response, though it is not clear whether it acts through the detoxifying action of the plasma
protein or through some beneficial effect of the protein *per se*, since small amounts remain
after the rinse. However, the amount of protein that can be left in the medium is sharply
restricted since, even with isogenous serum, the retina sticks to itself at protein levels
above 100 mg %, severely interfering with its diffusion exchange with the medium. Direct
comparison made between the medium shown in the Table and fresh human spinal fluid
revealed little difference in the electrical function of the retina, observed over a period of
several hours.

When no electrical recordings are to be made, incubations are performed in "boats"
(cf. Geiman, Anfinsen, McKee, Ormsbee and Ball, 1946) which provide a large surface of
medium for equilibration with the gas phase and which are rocked gently to effect continuous movement of the retina through the bathing fluid.

Two experimental systems have been used for making electrical recordings. In the first,
shown in Fig. 2, the entire retina is suspended by gross electrodes, one impaling the crushed

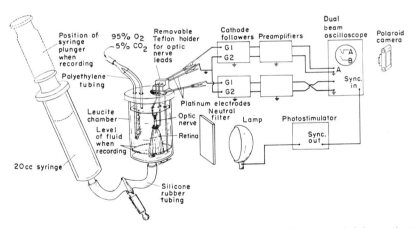

Fig. 2. Incubating and recording apparatus. Diagram shows retina suspended by optic nerve in
medium which can be withdrawn from the chamber by means of the syringe when electrical recording
is to be made. Gas mixture, saturated with water vapor, is admitted into chamber both above and below
the surface of the medium. (Reprinted from *J. Neurophysiol.* (1960), **23**, 676.)

end of the nerve segment and the other encircling the nerve at the disc. The light-evoked
compound action potential of the nerve is recorded between these electrodes (cf. Fig. 4A,
right). After lowering the medium by means of a syringe and with a third electrode contacting the region of the ora serrata via the lowered medium, a "retinal" potential can be
recorded between optic disc and ora serrata, with a geometric orientation that is tangential
to the surface of the retina (cf. Fig. 4A, *left*). This potential has many of the characteristics of the *a*-wave of the conventional ERG and of the P-III wave of Granit (cf. Ames

and Gurian, 1960; Pautler and Wilson, 1964). With microelectrodes introduced into the nerve, the spontaneous activity and light-evoked response of a single ganglion cell axon can be recorded (Ames and Gurian, 1961).

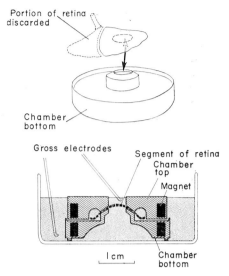

FIG. 3. Lucite "chamber" used to mount retina for electrical recordings. Upper drawing shows retina about to be positioned on lower half of chamber. Much of the retina including optic nerve stump (indicated by dotted portion in drawing) will be cut off and discarded before upper half of chamber is put in place.

Lower drawing shows cross-section of entire chamber with segment of retina in place. Level of medium and placement of platinum electrodes for recording electroretinogram are shown. (Reprinted from *Arch. Ophth.* (1963). **70**, 837.)

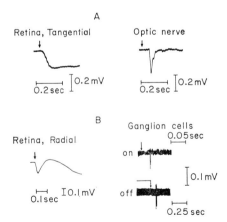

FIG. 4. Light-evoked responses recorded with gross electrodes directly from the retina (*upper left, lower left*) or from the optic nerve (*upper right*) or recorded with micro electrodes placed near ganglion cell bodies (*lower right*). Recordings in upper half of figure (A) obtained using chamber shown in Fig. 2; those in lower half (B) with chamber shown in Fig. 3. Arrows indicate time of short light flash; line-with-arrow indicates termination of prolonged light stimulus.

In a second preparation (cf. Fig. 3), still only partially developed, a disc of retina is fixed as a membrane separating two fluid-filled compartments in a fashion analogous to Ussing's treatment of frog skin (Ames and Gurian, 1963b). This has permitted recording of the ERG according to more conventional geometry (cf. Fig. 4B, *left*) and the relatively easy recording of single unit electrical responses with semi-microelectrodes placed near individual ganglion cells (cf. Fig. 4B, *right*). It also offers the potential, but as yet unexploited, opportunity of: measuring transretinal resistance, resting potential, and current flow; using small light patterns to stimulate, separately, inhibitory and excitatory receptor areas (e.g. Kuffler, 1953); measuring solute movements through the tissue; and making transretinal spectro-photometric measurements of the functioning tissue.

Other experimental systems have been described for *in vitro* maintenance of mammalian retina. Sickel, Lippmann, Haschke and Baumann (1960) have recorded light-evoked electrical responses from human retina suspended in a perfusion chamber between 2 layers of plastic mesh. Lucas (1962) has maintained guinea-pig retina for several days *in vitro*, Noell and Crapper (cf. Noell, 1963) have developed a modified *in vivo* preparation of rabbit retina through which they have measured resting potential, short-circuit current, and ion fluxes.

3. Results

Status of isolated retinas under control conditions

Retinas maintained *in vitro* for an hour or more appear to remain quite near to their normal physiological state. Their appearance under the light or electron microscope resembles closely that of retinas fixed *in vivo* (cf. Plate 1, from work of Webster and Ames, to be published). Their cellular contents of water and electrolytes remains close to *in vivo* levels in the control medium and there is little shift even during the procedure of isolation, though both water and electrolytes respond rapidly to experimental modifications of the medium (Ames and Hastings, 1956). Spontaneous and light-evoked electrical responses measured *in vitro* are similar to those obtained *in vivo* except that no c-wave is recorded—probably due to the absence from the preparation of the pigment epithelium (Ames and Gurian, 1960, 1963b).

The response of water and electrolytes in the retina to changes in medium osmolality

(These studies have been presented in detail [Ames, Isom and Nesbett, 1965].)

Retinal water and electrolytes were measured following incubation in a control medium or in one of four anisotonic media, and the amounts present in the cells were calculated using alternatively inulin, mannitol or Cl to label the extracellular water. As expected, total tissue water varied inversely with the osmolality of the medium. When total water was partitioned between an extracellular and an intracellular phase it was found that the intracellular phase responded as a perfect osmometer within the error of the method. Changes in the volume of the extracellular phase, though less marked, were in the same direction as the changes in the intracellular phase. Water movement was rapid, with a half-time of about 14 sec and attainment of a new steady state by 2 min. There was little subsequent change in the water distribution even when incubation in the anisotonic medium was extended to 2 hr. As osmolality was increased from 247 to 367 mOsm (by freezing point depression), there was a net movement of K into cells in spite of the increased concentration of intracellular K resulting from the exodus of water. Na moved in the opposite direction, to maintain approximately constant intracellular Na concentration in the face of the changing cell volume. There was little change, as a function of osmolality, in intracellular Cl—calculated with inulin as the extracellular label. At an osmolality between 247 (average cell volume 115% of normal) and 212 (average cell volume 133% of normal) the plasma membranes of at least some of the cells appeared to become altered by the cellular swelling, resulting in an appreciable exchange of intracellular K for Na and the probable entry of some inulin.

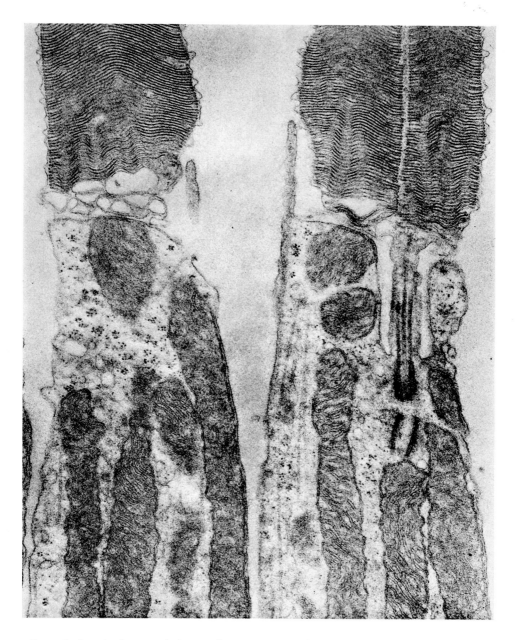

PLATE 1. Junction between the inner and outer segments of two receptor cells. ($\times$ 26,500) The retina was fixed in osmium tetroxide after incubation for 1 hr in control medium. (Electron micrograph by Dr. Henry deF Webster.)

Changes in the light-evoked electrical response of isolated retina during and after deprivation of O_2, glucose, or both.

(These studies have been presented in detail [Ames and Gurian, 1963a].)

The apparatus shown in Fig. 2 was used in these experiments. Most of them were performed at 30°C. The light-evoked compound action potential recorded from the optic nerve failed rapidly in the absence of O_2, falling to 50% of normal in one minute and disappearing entirely within 4 min (Fig. 5). These changes were completely reversible even after 60 min of deprivation (Fig. 6). Medium glucose could be reduced

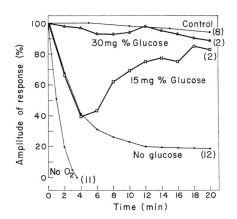

Fig. 5. Amplitude of light-evoked compound action potentials recorded from optic nerve and plotted relative to control response recorded at zero time. Various curves show change in amplitude during incubation in control medium and in media containing normal glucose, but no O_2; normal O_2 but no glucose; normal O_2 and two intermediate levels of glucose as shown. (Reprinted, slightly modified, from *J. Neurophysiol.* (1963). **26**, 617.)

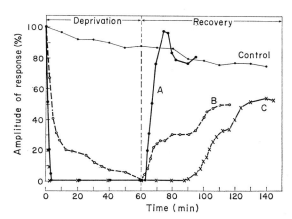

Fig. 6. Amplitude of light-evoked response in optic nerve plotted as in Fig. 5. The three curves show changes during and after 1 hr of deprivation at 30°C, of O_2 alone (A), glucose alone (B), or both O_2 and glucose (C). Fine line at top shows behavior of controls over same period.

to 30 mg % (1·7mM) without apparent effect, (Fig. 5) but, when glucose was removed altogether, the response recorded from the nerve began to fail immediately, falling to 40% of normal in 4 min and to 0 in 60 min (Figs. 5 and 6). With glucose levels at 15 mg %, function failed for 4 min as rapidly as with no glucose present, but the tissue then seemed to adapt to these low concentrations of glucose, and function returned almost to normal levels over the course of the next 16 min (Fig. 5). Glucose deprivation was much less reversible than O_2 deprivation, with a significant degree of irreversible damage occurring within 10 min and increasing thereafter (Fig. 6). When both O_2 and glucose were removed simultaneously, function failed rapidly and recovery was delayed, but was finally at least as complete as following glucose deprivation alone (Fig. 6). Increasing the temperature from 30° to 37° C reduced the period of combined deprivation that could be reversibly sustained by about a factor of 3. The short-latency, prolonged, potential shift recorded directly from the retina was more resistant to the deprivations than the light-evoked response in the nerve.

The ultrastructure of retinas deprived of both oxygen and glucose at 37°C.

(These studies have been presented in detail and are now in press [Webster and Ames, 1965].)

Deprivation of oxygen and glucose for 10 min produced marked mitochondrial enlargement with separation of cristae in the receptor cell inner segments. Less swelling occurred in mitochondria of the bipolar cells, ganglion cells and myelinated axons. Focal dilatation of Golgi membranes and endoplasmic reticulum cisternae was also apparent. More severe swelling of these organelles was present after 20 min, while 30 min of the combined deprivation resulted in multiple discontinuities in the membranes of cell organelles and nuclei, as well as those bounding cell surfaces.

If oxygen and glucose were resupplied after 10 or 20 min of deprivation, the alterations in cell organelles showed a considerable degree of reversibility. After 30 min, however, the changes had become almost completely irreversible. There was a general parallelism between the reversibility of the morphologic changes and the recovery of electrophysiologic function, as studied previously under similar conditions.

4. Discussion

As a consequence of its geometry and vascular supply, the retina is particularly suited to study *in vitro*. The evidence presently available, based on morphologic, chemical and electro-physiological studies, indicates that isolated retina can be maintained in a condition closely approximating its normal physiological state for a period of several hours. It is often possible to introduce experimental variables and to make measurements on the isolated tissue with greater ease and precision than would be possible *in vivo*.

The studies cited represent early efforts to realize some of the advantages offered by this preparation. It seems particularly fortunate that a tissue so well suited to study *in vitro* should incorporate phenomena of such general biological interest as photoreception, transduction of the photochemical event into a neural event, and rather complex neural processing of the information received.

REFERENCES

Ames, A., III and Gurian, B. S. (1960). *J. Neurophysiol.* **23**, 676.
Ames, A., III and Gurian, B. S. (1961). *Science* **133** (3466), 1767.
Ames, A., III and Gurian, B. S. (1963a). *J. Neurophysiol.* **26**, 617.
Ames, A., III and Gurian, B. S. (1963b). *Arch. Ophthal.* **70**, 837.
Ames, A., III and Hastings, A. B. (1956). *J. Neurophysiol.* **19**, 201.
Ames, A., III, Isom, J. B. and Nesbett, F. B. (1965). *J. Physiol.* **177**, 246.
Geiman, Q. M., Anfinsen, C. B., McKee, R. W., Ormsbee, R. A. and Ball, E. G. (1946). *J. exp. Med.* **84**, 583.

Kuffler, S. W. (1953). *J. Neurophysiol.* **16**, 37.

Lucas, D. R. (1962). *Vision Res.* **2**, 35.

Noell, W. K. (1963). *J. opt. soc. Am.* **53**, 36.

Paulter, E. L. and Wilson, R. A. (1963). *Vision Res.* **3**, 507.

Sickel, W., Lippmann, H. G., Haschke, W. and Baumann, Ch. (1960). *Elektrogramm der umstrom-
ten menschlichen Retina.* 63. Tagg. d. Dtsch. Ophthalmolog.-Ges., Berlin, pp. 316-318.

Webster, H. deF. and Ames, A., III (1965). *J. Cell Biol.* in press.

DISCUSSION

DR. COLE remarked that he had found a similar effect of anoxia on the standing potential of the ciliary body, and that, as in the case of the retina, there was a rapid recovery on return to oxygen. He thought it might be of interest to study electrolyte changes in an isotonic medium of low sodium content, these precise conditions not having been studied by Dr. Ames. This could be achieved by substituting mannitol for some of the sodium. He was particularly interested in whether the observed effects were due to changes in general tonicity or to a specific ion.

DR. AMES, in reference to this question, said that little difference was apparent in media made hypertonic with sodium or mannitol, which was indirect evidence that the nature of the ion was not important in this respect.

DR. AMES agreed in principle with DR. COLE's comment that there was a straightforward relationship between oxygen consumption and increases of electrical potential and short-circuit current (indicating an increase in sodium transport).

PROFESSOR COHEN queried the 'rebound' effect of the 'medium-low' glucose concentration (15 mg %) and suggested that this might result from a build-up of lactic acid in one part of the retina which was used subsequently as a fuel elsewhere. It could be, he added, that a time interval was required to build up this energy source and hence the delay in return to normal activity. DR. AMES stressed that this would not apply to the medium, in which dilution would annul the effects of any accumulated substrate. The question of accumulation *within* the tissue remained a possibility, however.

DR. PEDLER asked DR. AMES whether he considered the alignment of the mitochondria to be abnormal after 10 min of deprivation. DR. AMES explained that he was not suggesting a difference of alignment at this time but that the mitochondria became swollen.

DR. KEEN commented on the fact that he felt that the inability of pyruvate to support electrical activity, as shown by Dr. Ames, cast doubt on the possibility that lactate accumulation played any role in this phenomenon of recovery.

In reply to questions from DR. ARDEN, DR. AMES explained that he had not as yet investigated the presence of a resting potential in his second preparation, although he was in process of assembling the necessary equipment. DR. ARDEN asked also whether all the recovery curves shown represented optic nerve responses or whether some were ERGs—he felt that the latter could be more readily correlated with the electron-micrographs of the receptor organelles. DR. AMES replied that those he had shown were optic nerve responses, although he had studied ERGs using the first experimental technique in which potentials recorded tangentially from the retina seemed to correlate quite well with the P-III of Granit. He had found these to be more resistant to deprivation than the optic nerve responses, and they also showed an earlier recovery, but nevertheless, they showed the same changes qualitatively. He remarked that the changes in the ERG were less consistent in these preparations than changes in the nerve response.

Dr. Arden also queried the recovery of dark adaptation in the isolated retina, and the increase in sensitivity through which the retina changed when it was dark adapted. Dr. Ames said that he felt that previously published work (Ames and Gurion, 1960, Fig. 9) showed evidence of re-adaptation to the dark although there was no quantitative evidence of the fate of rhodopsin in the tissues. He added that retinas from dark adapted rabbits showed red coloration and bleached on illumination. If, subsequently, they were incubated in the dark there was no apparent subjective return of colour. Yet there was a return in the amplitude of the optic nerve response. Dr. Ames agreed that it was difficult to reconcile these phenomena and account for this.

Dr. Bridges mentioned that a colleague of his in Miami, Dr. Hamasaki, had observed the same effect in isolated frog retinas, and again, there was no evidence of pigment regeneration. Professor Cohen added that he felt the problem was not so much one of visual purple and light adaptation, but of the pigment and excitation. It was obvious that visual purple must be present unless one conceded that it was not necessary for this last process!

Professor Noell referred to similar experiments conducted in his laboratory by Hanawa, again using the retina of the frog. One of the most striking features, he added, was the markedly adverse effect of sodium depletion on the ERG, the whole response being reduced considerably. He mentioned that many years ago when he had been studying the effect of anoxia *in vivo*, he had found that the disappearance of the optic nerve response was due to a failure in the ganglion cells, any failure of visual cell organization being secondary as regards the time course of events.

Professor Noell felt it was important to stress that oxygen availability might differ considerably between *in vitro* and *in vivo* conditions, and that this might contribute to the 'abnormal' reaction of the isolated retina. If one applied the classical Warburg formula it could be seen that the vitreous could do little more than supply oxygen to a depth of about 5 μ in the retina.

Professor Noell also queried the disappearance of the cristae from the mitochondria during glucose deprivation as well as the reversal of this effect. Dr. Ames speaking on behalf of his colleague Dr. Webster said that he understood that the mitochondria of the inner segments showed the greatest facility for reversal of damage following deprivation of glucose; the mitochondria of the axons appeared to have least potential for such recovery.

Professor Potts asked how one could reconcile the electrical response of the isolated retina with the effects of clinical detachment. The response was lost rapidly in these circumstances, but could be restored by re-attachment. Dr. Ames explained that he felt that the fall in ambient oxygen resulting from separation of the choroid from the retina would be sufficient to induce loss of function. This was, nevertheless, reversible. He thought that there was quite a margin between the critical level required for viability and that required for normal functioning.

Dr. Arden agreed that in experimental detachment the activity of the retina could be restored after quite long periods.

Glycogen Synthesis by the Rat Retina*

Shinji Kurimoto,† Frank W. Newell and Tibor G. Farkas

Eye Research Laboratories, The University of Chicago, Chicago 37, Illinois, U.S.A.

Uniformly labeled D-[^{14}C]glucose 1-phosphate was incorporated into glycogen when incubated with retinal homogenates of normal and alloxan-diabetic rats. Incorporation of D-[^{14}C]glucose 1-phosphate into retinal glycogen of alloxan-diabetic rats showed a significant increase in comparison with retinal glycogen of normal rats.

The excess of glycogen in the alloxan-diabetic rat was not a result of an increase in phosphorylase-b activity inasmuch as there was no significant change in the phosphorylase-a/phosphorylase-b ratio in the normal and alloxan-diabetic rat retina. The rate of incorporation of uniformly labeled D-[^{14}C]glucose 1-P into glycogen was linear for the first 60 min in both the normal and diabetic rat retina.

1. Introduction

It has been reported previously (Kurimoto and Newell, 1963) that the retinas of alloxan-diabetic rats show increased glycogen synthesis *in vitro* and accumulation of glycogen *in vivo*. It has also been suggested that the accumulation of glycogen might be due either to an increase in the activity of UDPG‡-glycogen transferase or to an increase in phosphorylase-b activity. However, increased activity of UDPG-glycogen transferase of retinas of alloxan-diabetic rats could not be demonstrated (Newell and Kurimoto, 1963) histochemically.

This study was undertaken in order to evaluate the phosphorylase-b activity of the retinas of alloxan-diabetic rats by radioactive tracer methods.

2. Materials and Methods

Male albino Sprague-Dawley rats, weighing 180–212 g, received 20 mg of alloxan per 100 g of body weight subcutaneously. The animals were fed standard Purina rat chow. Twenty-three of the animals were sacrificed 168–179 days after the alloxan administration (average 173 days). An equal number of untreated rats were maintained for the same period of time as normal controls.

The urine of the alloxan diabetic rats repeatedly showed 4+ reduction when tested with 'tape', while the urine of the control animals was negative. Before sacrifice, the animals were fasted for 24 hr. At this time the body weight of the diabetic rats varied between 95 and 210 g (average weight 158 g) while the weight of the control animals fluctuated between 330 and 500 g (average weight 396 g).

The blood glucose level of the diabetic animals at the time of sacrifice varied between 204 and 949 mg/100 ml (average 379 mg/100 ml) while the blood sugar of the control animals was between 78 and 114 mg/100 ml (average 92 mg/100 ml). All the diabetic animals had cataracts and none was present in the normal controls.

The eyes were enucleated, placed on ice and incised circumferentially at the equator. The vitreous was removed and the retina was dissected free. The retinas of each animal

* This work was supported in part by the United States Public Health Service Sensory Disease Program Project grant no. NB-03358.

† Fight-for-Sight Fellow of the National Council to Combat Blindness, Inc., New York, N.Y., U.S.A.

‡ Abbreviations used: UDPG, uridine diphosphate glucose; PR, phosphate remover.

were homogenized* in 4·5 ml of ice-cold 0·02 M NaF-0·001 M ethylene diamine-tetra-acetic acid (EDTA). The NaF-EDTA solution was adjusted to pH 6·0 in order to minimize the removal of glucose 1-phosphate by phosphoglucomutase (Cori, Illingworth and Keller, 1955).

A 2·0 ml aliquot of the homogenates was transferred to a test tube and 1·0 ml of 4·2% glycogen in 0·02 M NaF-0·001 M EDTA, pH 6·0 and 1·0 ml of $4·2 \times 10^{-3}$ M 5'-adenylic acid (AMP) in 0·02 M NaF-0·001 M EDTA, pH 6·0 was added. In a further 2·0 ml aliquot, 1·0 ml of 0·02 M NaF-0·001 M EDTA was substituted for the AMP. The tubes were covered with Parafilm and prewarmed for 33 min in a shaking water bath (100 osc/min) at 37°C. The reaction was started by adding 200 μl (0·01 μc) of $2·95 \times 10^{-6}$ M uniformly labeled [^{14}C]glucose 1-phosphate in 0·02 M NaF-0·001 M EDTA, pH 6·0 to the incubation mixture. The reaction was permitted to proceed for 60 min at 37°C in the shaking water bath. At the end of 60 min two separate 2·0 ml aliquots were removed from the incubation mixture and the reaction was terminated by the addition of an equal volume of ice-cold 10% trichloroacetic acid (TCA). The solution was centrifuged and the clear supernatant decanted. The precipitate was washed with 2·0 ml of ice-cold 5% TCA. After centrifugation the supernate was decanted. The washed precipitate was dissolved in 1·0 N NaOH for protein determination (Lowry, Rosebrough, Farr and Randall, 1951).

The original supernatant and the washing were combined and an equal volume of 100% ethanol was added in order to precipitate the glycogen. The precipitated glycogen was removed by centrifugation (4100 rev/min for 30 min) and dissolved in 5·0 ml of 5% TCA. The glycogen was reprecipitated from solution by the addition of 5·0 ml of 100% ethanol. The precipitate was again separated by centrifugation and then dissolved in 5·0 ml of hot water. The glycogen was again precipitated with 5·0 ml of 100% ethanol. After centrifugation, the last supernatant was counted in a scintillation counter in order to detect any radioactivity. The precipitated glycogen was placed in a hot water bath in order to remove all traces of adherent ethanol. The purified glycogen was hydrolyzed by heating it with 2·0 ml of 0·6 N H_2SO_4 for 3 hr in a boiling water bath. The tubes were covered in order to prevent loss of water by evaporation during hydrolysis.

The glucose solution was diluted with an equal volume of distilled water to prevent turbidity when the nondiluted solution was mixed with the scintillator solution. The scintillator solution consisted of 42 ml of Liquifluor and 100 g of naphthalene in 1000 ml of dioxane. 1·0 ml of the diluted glucose solution was mixed with 15·0 ml of scintillator solution and counted in a Packard Tricarb scintillation counter (efficiency of 66·9%). At the end of the counting 100 μl of $2·95 \times 10^{-6}$ M uniformly labeled [^{14}C]glucose 1-phosphate (s.a. = 16·7 mc/mmole) was added to both the sample and control vials in order to ascertain that there was no difference in the quenching effect between sample and control. The results were expressed as counts per minute per milligram of protein per hour (ct/min per mg/hr).

For the time course incorporation study, instead of 2·0 ml aliquots 1·0 ml was removed at 15 min intervals for a total of 60 min. Duplicate samples could not be taken in this study. The purified glycogen was hydrolyzed by 1·0 ml of 0·6 N H_2SO_4 instead of 2·0 ml but the other procedures were based on previously described methods (Illingworth, Kronfeld and Brown, 1960; Cowgill and Pardee, 1957).

3. Results

The results of the incorporation study are presented in Table I. There is a significant increase in the incorporation of uniformly labeled D-[^{14}C]glucose 1-phosphate into glycogen of the retinas of alloxan-diabetic rats when compared with normal controls.

Incorporation of glucose 1-phosphate without AMP represents phosphorylase-a activity, while incorporation in the presence of AMP is due to total phosphorylase

* Microchemical Specialties Company Homogenizer, 1825 Eastshore Highway, Berkeley 10, Calif., U.S.A.

activity. The phosphorylase-a/total phosphorylase activity ratio was 56·71% in the normal controls and 55·71% in the retinas of alloxan-diabetic rats. The difference in these ratios is not significant statistically. Neither was there any difference in the phosphorylase-a/phosphorylase-b ratio of normal and alloxan-diabetic rat retinas (1·28 vs 1·26, respectively).

TABLE I

Incorporation of the uniformly labeled D-[¹⁴C]glucose 1-phosphate into glycogen of retinas of normal and alloxan-diabetic rats

Animals	Radioactivity of retinal glycogen cts/min per mg of protein/hr	
	Without AMP	With AMP
Normal	2893 ± 101·6*	5130 ± 100·4*
Diabetic	3554 ± 140·3*	6380 ± 134·4*
P	<0·001	<0·001

* Standard error.
Each figure is based on 23 separate determinations.

The incorporation of uniformly labeled D-[¹⁴C]glucose 1-phosphate into glycogen was linear for the first 60 min in the retinas of both normal and alloxan-diabetic rats (see Fig. 1).

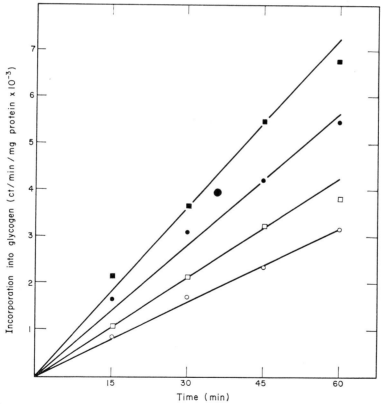

FIG. 1. Time course of incorporation of uniformly labeled D-[¹⁴C]glucose 1-phosphate into glycogen by normal and alloxan-diabetic rat retinas. Each point represents the average of 11 rats.
●, Normal rat (+AMP); ○, normal rat (−AMP); ■, diabetic rat (+AMP); □, diabetic rat (−AMP).

c

4. Discussion

It is well known that glycogen exists in tissues in an "extractable" and "residual" form. This study concerns itself only with the extractable form of glycogen. It cannot be assumed that the incorporation of ^{14}C-labeled glucose 1-phosphate represents a measure of glycogen synthesis. Although incorporation represents the molecules that have been converted into glycogen unchanged and have not undergone any degradative process, a correlation has been established between incorporation and the net result of glycogen synthesis and degradation (Figueroa and Pfeifer, 1962). Glycogen is synthesized *in vitro* from glucose 1-phosphate either by phosphorylase or by UDPG-glycogen transferase. The results of this study indicate the phosphorylase activity only. The data of this study confirmed the previous finding of increased glycogen synthesis by phosphorylase in alloxan-diabetic rat retina *in vitro*. Phosphorylase-a is an enzyme which can act with or without the presence of AMP, while phosphorylase-b requires AMP for its action. The incorporation data obtained in the absence of AMP refer to the phosphorylase-a activity while the phosphorylase-b activity can be calculated by difference. Kurachi (1963) reported that the activity of phosphorylase-a in retinal homogenates of rabbits or hens was a quarter of the total phosphorylase activity; that is, phosphorylase-b is three times as active as phosphorylase-a in the retina. In the present study, phosphorylase-b activity was about 44% of the total phosphorylase activity. Because many tissues contain an enzyme, PR, which converts phosphorylase-a into phosphorylase-b, the action of this enzyme must be prevented if accurate determination of phosphorylase-a and -b is desired. The EDTA-NaF solution used in this study prevented the action of PR enzyme and that of a specific kinase which is known to change the relative proportions of phosphorylase-a and -b. It has been demonstrated that in tissue homogenates made with EDTA-NaF, the ratio of phosphorylase-a and -b remained constant for a period of several days (Illingworth et al., 1960). The phosphorylase-a/phosphorylase-b ratio was not significantly different in retinas of normal and alloxan-diabetic rats. *In vivo* glycogen accumulation in retinas of alloxan-diabetic rats therefore was not the result of an increase in phosphorylase-b.

Since glycogen is also synthesized by the UDPG-glycogen transferase system, the observed *in vivo* glycogen accumulation might be due to an increase in the activity of this enzyme system. We have failed, however, to demonstrate unequivocally increased UDPG-glycogen transferase activity in retinas of alloxan-diabetic rats using histochemical techniques. Bo and Smith (1963) suggested that glycogen synthesis using glucose 1-phosphate as the substrate was catalyzed by the phosphorylase system and not through the UDPG pathways in the uterus of oophorectomized or oophorectomized-hormone treated rats because no UDPG-glycogen transferase could be demonstrated in the uterus. Bueding (1962) observed that there were greater similarities among phosphorylases of the same tissue in different species than between two different tissues. Hutchinson and Kuwabara (1963) reported that the phosphorylase content of the retinas of a variety of animals was remarkably constant while the glycogen content of this tissue varied from species to species. Currently, experiments are in progress in our laboratory in order to measure the UDPG glycogen transferase activity directly in the retinas of alloxan-diabetic rats.

ACKNOWLEDGMENTS

The authors are indebted to Miss Yi-Min Shao for her skilful technical assistance. Grateful acknowledgment is made to Vera Glocklin, Ph.D. (University of Chicago) for her valuable advice.

REFERENCES

Bo, W. J. and Smith, M. S. (1963). *Proc. Soc. exp. Biol. Med.* **113**, 812.
Bueding, E. (1962). *Fed. Proc.* **21**, 1039.
Cori, G. T., Illingworth, B. and Keller, P. J. (1955). In *Methods in Enzymology*, ed. by Colowick, S. P. and Kaplan, N. O. Academic Press, New York.
Cowgill, R. W. and Pardee, A. B. (1957). *Experiments in Biological Research Techniques*. John Wiley and Sons, Inc., New York.
Figueroa, E. and Pfeifer, A. (1962). *Arch. Biochim. Biophys. Acta* **99**, 357.
Hutchinson, T. B. and Kuwabara, T. (1962). *Arch. Ophth.* **68**, 538.
Illingworth, B., Kronfeld, R. and Brown, D. H. (1960). *Biochim. biophys. Acta* **42**, 486.
Kurachi, Y. (1963). *Acta Soc. ophthal. jap.* **67**, 1241.
Kurimoto, S. and Newell, F. W. (1963). *Invest. Ophth.* **2**, 24.
Lowry, O. H., Rosebrough, N. J., Farr, A. L. and Randall, R. J. (1951). *J. biol. Chem.* **193**, 265.
Newell, F. W. and Kurimoto, S. (1963). *Br. J. Ophthal.* **47**, 596.

DISCUSSION

Dr. KUWABARA commented on the difficulty of demonstrating UDPG synthetase activity in whole tissue preparations. He had found the same problem but had noted that fairly high synthetase activity could be demonstrated in areas of broken tissue or at cut edges. He wondered, therefore, whether this might merely be a problem of substrate permeability.

PROFESSOR NEWELL emphasized that the radioactive studies were carried out on homogenized tissue in which injury was ignored as a factor; he felt that one would have to experiment with the medium if one wished to promote uptake. Certainly, he added, the normal preparation used for histochemical demonstration of UDPG, although quite successful in the rectus muscle for example, was not able to demonstrate uptake in the retina. A cut-edge phenomenon occurred, but nevertheless, it was far more difficult to demonstrate the UDPG system than that of phosphorylase. He was particularly intrigued by reports—on uterus muscle for example—that although no UDPG systems could be shown, glycogen synthesis occurred, apparently even *in vivo*, making use of the phosphorylase system.

Dr. KEEN queried whether the experiments described demonstrated increased glycogen synthesis or increased enzyme capacity. PROFESSOR NEWELL pointed out that the older methods used for the demonstration of glycogen were not satisfactory. Recent histochemical techniques employed enzymatic synthesis, and it was very difficult to decide whether these indicated increased glycogen deposition, or enzymatic potential, a point that was discussed at length by the meeting.

Dr. EVERSON PEARSE pointed out during this discussion that from the standpoint of the histochemical technique, phosphorylase would produce an unbranched glycogen staining completely differently from the normal branched variety. Therefore no control was necessary. The UDPG system, he added, was quite different, and the difficulty of control did arise. He felt it was possible that the glycogen was being destroyed as rapidly as it was formed.

Relationships between Visual Function and Metabolism

L. H. Cohen* and W. K. Noell

*Department of Biochemistry, University of Manitoba, Winnipeg, Canada,
and Department of Physiology, University of Buffalo, Buffalo, N.Y., U.S.A.*

The visual cell has an unusually high glycolysis and an unusually high respiration. The respiration can be used almost entirely for the oxidation of carbohydrate by the citric acid cycle. There is also a high capacity for the pentose phosphate path but, *in vitro* at least, it is limited by the availability of electron acceptors. The systems for glucose oxidation and glycolysis are separated in such a way as to favor independent activity. Since the system for glucose oxidation is concentrated close to the site of light absorption, it is suggested that glucose oxidation may be specialized for the support of the initial events of vision and that the outer limb might be a light-activated electron transport agent. Upon illumination, a portion of the electron transport would occur through the outer limb to generate chemical and electrical signals. The possible nature of these signals, the metabolic paths involved in their production, and the mechanism of light activation are discussed.

When a tissue is found to have unusual metabolic properties, it is a reasonable assumption that these properties are involved in the special function of that tissue. The retina is one such tissue. As Warburg showed many years ago (Warburg, Posener and Negelein, 1924; Warburg, 1927) the isolated retina has three unusual properties: it converts glucose to lactic acid with prodigious speed; it consumes oxygen more rapidly than other tissues; and the formation of lactic acid is rapid even in the presence of oxygen, aerobic glycolysis† being only about one-third less than anaerobic glycolysis.

However, it is not easy to guess the relation between these properties and visual function. The retina contains several cell types, each with its own role in vision, and it is important to know which cell types possess a given metabolic property. There are several approaches to this information. One procedure used by several investigators has been the histochemical and cytochemical study of the location of individual enzymes. These techniques have furnished much valuable evidence, indicating that several enzymes are not uniformly distributed among the various cell types. As yet, these methods are limited to a few enzymes and in some cases are not quantitative, so that it is highly desirable to supplement this information with other types of evidence in order to learn about the sites of integrated metabolic pathways in the retina. We have therefore tried several other approaches. First, we have studied the young retina at various ages in order to learn whether the development of these exceptional metabolic activities is associated with the differentiation of specific structures of the retina. Second, we have examined the kinetics of respiration and glycolysis of the retina for manifestations of compartmentation of metabolism. Respiration and glycolysis usually influence each other if they are in the same compartment: if one depresses respiration by anaerobiosis, then glycolysis is stimulated (Pasteur effect); if one depresses glycolysis by withholding glucose from the medium, respiration is stimulated (Crabtree effect). The Crabtree effect has been observed only with tissues

---

* Present address: Institute for Cancer Research, Fox Chase, Philadelphia, Pa., U.S.A.
† In this presentation glycolysis denotes the formation of lactic acid from carbohydrates.

which have a high glycolytic capacity, so one might expect it to be obtained with the retina. Another, highly desirable, approach is to separate the different cell types of the retina. It is possible to obtain retinas from which the visual cell layer has been removed, by taking advantage of the unusual sensitivity of the visual cells to iodo-acetate. Several years ago (Noell, 1951) it was found that the intravenous administration of a small dose of iodoacetate immediately blocks the electroretinogram for several hours. Slightly larger doses produce complete destruction and resorption of the rods within 2 weeks after administration of the poison, leaving a retina lacking the visual cell layer. From studies of the metabolism of these retinas one should be able to learn something about the visual cells.

These approaches are largely indirect and some of the interpretations rest upon assumptions that are not completely proven, but, as will be seen, the results fit into a fairly consistent picture.

The development study (Cohen, 1957; Cohen and Noell, 1960) showed that the metabolism of the rabbit retina is not so active at birth as it is in the adult, and that shortly after birth striking changes occur, particularly in respiration, as shown by the upper curve of Fig. 1. The respiratory rate at birth is very low and increases several-

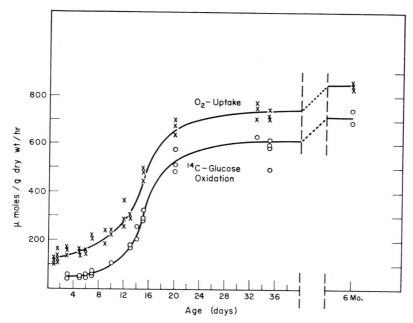

Fig. 1. Respiration and glucose oxidation of rabbit retina in relation to postnatal age. Medium was calcium-free Krebs-Ringer-phosphate buffer containing 20 mM uniformly labelled [^{14}C]glucose; incubation was for 65 min.

fold* between the ages of 8 and 20 days, with the steepest rise between 12 and 20 days. Over 95% of the increase in oxygen uptake is accounted for by the oxidation of glucose to carbon dioxide, shown in the lower curve. We have also found (see Noell, 1958a,b) that just preceding this change in respiratory rate there is a substantial increase

* In these measurements calcium ion was omitted from the medium. The increase in respiration during development would not appear as large if calcium ion were included, since respiration of the adult retina is depressed 50% by calcium ions, whereas the young retina is only slightly affected (Cohen and Noell, 1959, 1960).

(70–80%) in anaerobic glycolysis, which occurs between the 4th and 10th day after birth, and that there is a doubling of aerobic glycolysis between the 4th and 20th day after birth. A similar increase in respiration and glycolysis occurs in the rat retina (Graymore, 1959, 1960) and mouse retina (Noell, this Symposium).

The rate of oxidation of glucose to carbon dioxide by the adult retina shown here greatly exceeds that reported for other animal tissues, including brain slices (Wenner and Weinhouse, 1956; Di Pietro and Weinhouse, 1959). What pathways are responsible for this extremely rapid glucose oxidation? To answer this question we studied the fates of the various carbon atoms of glucose under a wide variety of experimental conditions (Cohen and Noell, 1958, 1959, 1960). This study showed that the adult retina possesses high capacities for both the citric acid cycle and the pentose phosphate path. Under ordinary conditions of *in vitro* incubation, however, (aerobic, no pyruvate or electron transport mediators added to the medium) the pentose phosphate path was found to be limited by the availability of electron acceptors, and the oxidation of glucose carbon to carbon dioxide was carried out almost entirely by the citric acid cycle, with the possible exception of the carbon at position 1 of the glucose molecule.*

Of all the alterations in metabolism found to occur postnatally, therefore, the most pronounced is the increase in glucose oxidation by the citric acid cycle. The oxidation of carbon-6 of glucose to carbon dioxide by this path was 20–30 times more rapid in the adult than in the young retina (Cohen and Noell, 1960). The timing of this increase is very interesting. It closely parallels the appearance and increase of the electroretinogram and the formation and growth of the inner and outer limbs of the rods (Noell and Cohen, 1957; Noell, 1958a, b). Does this mean that the newly acquired glucose oxidation resides entirely in these sensory organelles? In order to get more evidence about this matter, we have studied rabbit retinas lacking visual cells (see Noell, 1958a, b). Dr. Graymore and his colleagues have independently carried out similar studies with the rat. Graymore and Tansley (1959) measured anaerobic glycolysis of retinas of which the visual cells had been destroyed by iodoacetate poisoning *in vivo*, and found it to be half that of the normal retina. They also studied retinas, lacking visual cells, from rats with *retinitis pigmentosa*, and found that both anaerobic glycolysis and respiration had about half the normal rates (Graymore, 1960; Graymore, Tansley and Kerly, 1959). These results indicated that respiration and glycolysis were much greater in the visual cells than in the rest of the retina, and that the visual cells were principally responsible for the marked increase in both of these activities which occurs in the rat retina during the first few weeks after birth. These investigators also pointed out an alternative explanation, that the metabolic activities of the non-visual cell layers might be lower than normal after destruction of the visual cells.

Our studies of the rabbit retina led us to similar conclusions. We have measured glucose oxidation as well as respiration, and the results are shown in Table I. The

---

* The evidence indicated that at least 10% of the C-1 oxidation occurred by way of the pentose phosphate path under ordinary conditions, judging from the difference in the amount of CO_2 formed from C-1 and from C-6 of glucose. However, we could not exclude the possibility that, in addition, some glucose could pass through the pentose path and then, by way of the Embden-Meyerhof path, enter the citric acid cycle. In this way C-1 would be converted to carbon dioxide in the pentose phosphate path and the other carbons would be oxidized in the citric acid cycle without evidence of a difference between C-1 and C-6 oxidation.

Experiments in which special conditions were employed to detect the pentose path revealed that the capacity for C-1 oxidation by this path was very great in both the young and adult retina and was twice as high in the adult retina as in the young retina (Cohen and Noell, 1958, 1959, 1960). A large capacity for the pentose phosphate path has also been reported for ox retina (Futterman and Kinoshita, 1959).

respiration and glucose oxidation are substantially lower in the retinas lacking visual cells than in the normal retinas, suggesting that in the rabbit retina too the visual cells have an even higher activity than the rest of the retina. However, unlike the case

TABLE I

Respiration, glucose oxidation and Crabtree effect in young retina, adult retina and visual-cell-less retina (from IAA treated rabbits)

Retina from:	O_2 uptake (glucose present) mμmoles/ mg dry wt/hr	Glucose carbon oxidized to CO_2		Crabtree effect
		mμatoms/ mg dry wt/hr	% of O_2 consumed	
7 day rabbit	156	54	35%	32% I
Adult rabbit	410	280	67%	10% I
Adult lacking visual cells	362	200	55%	25% I
Visual cells*	460	360	78%	No I (6% stim.)

Retinas were incubated in Krebs-Ringer-phosphate medium containing Ca^{++} with or without 20 mM uniformly-labelled [^{14}C]glucose. For measurements of the Crabtree effect, comparisons between glucose present and absent were performed on two retinas of the same animal. I = inhibition.

* Calculated on the basis of two assumptions: (a) the metabolism of non-visual cell layers is un-affected by destruction of visual cells; and (b) visual cell layer constitutes 50% of dry weight of normal retina.

of the rat, the respiration (and glucose oxidation) of the non-visual cell layers is much higher than that of the young rabbit, suggesting that the post-natal increase in glucose oxidation shown in Fig. 1 is not restricted entirely to the visual cells, although it would appear to be more pronounced in the visual cells than in the other cell layers.

Measurement of the Crabtree effect in these retinas provided some interesting information. This effect in the adult retina, although consistently observed, is very small. When the visual cells are missing, however, the Crabtree effect is substantial and calculation on the basis of the assumptions shown in Table I indicates that the visual cells may have no Crabtree effect at all. We should emphasize that this calculated value is approximate, but it does suggest that respiration of the visual cell is not in contact with a high-capacity glycolytic system. Yet, when we measured glycolysis, retinas lacking visual cells were found to have the same glycolysis (per mg dry weight) as the intact retina (Table II), indicating that the visual cell, as in the case

TABLE II

Anaerobic glycolysis and Pasteur effect

	Lactate formed† anaerobically mμmoles/mg dry wt/hr	Lactate in N_2 Lactate in air
7-day rabbit	1470	1·5
Adult rabbit	2450	1·3
Adult lacking visual cells	2600	1·8
"Visual cells"*	2400	1

The medium was Krebs-Ringer-phosphate buffer containing Ca^{++}.

* Calculated according to the assumptions shown in Table I.

† Measured during a 10-min. incubation period, these values approach initial rates.

of the rat, has a very high glycolytic capacity, although in this case not higher than the rest of the retina. When the Pasteur effect in these retinas was measured it was found that the retinas lacking visual cells had a more substantial Pasteur effect than the whole retina, and calculation indicated that to account for this the visual cell would have to have no Pasteur effect at all (last column, Table II).

Thus, our results and those of Graymore and his colleagues, while differing in some respects, both indicate that the visual cells possess unusually high respiration and glycolysis. The apparent absence of the Pasteur and Crabtree effects in these cells would therefore suggest that respiration and glycolysis are somehow separated from each other. Moreover, the respiratory system of the visual cells would seem to be specially suited for the oxidation of glucose, since the calculated glucose oxidation accounts for almost 80% of the respiration of the visual cell, and only 55% of the respiration of the non-visual cell layers.

These conclusions, although consistent with the data, are clearly based upon a number of assumptions. However, there are several reasons for believing them to be essentially correct. First, they agree very well with available histological and histochemical evidence. The visual cell has been found to be very rich in hexokinase and phosphofructokinase (Lowry, Roberts, Schulz, Clow and Clark, 1961). Since the

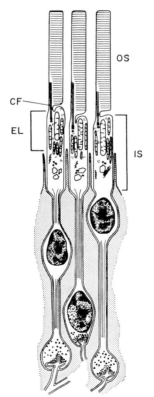

FIG. 2. The visual cells of the rabbit. OS, outer segments; IS, inner segments; EL, ellipsoid region; CF, ciliary filaments (modified from Noell, 1959).

reactions catalysed by these enzymes are believed to be rate-controlling for the Embden-Meyerhof path (Lardy and Parks, 1956; Lowry, Passonneau, Harselberger and Schutz, 1964; Rose and O'Connell, 1964) this would appear to confirm the view that glucose metabolism is very active in the visual cell. All of the mitochondria of the rabbit visual cell are clustered at one end of the inner limb, the ellipsoid region, leaving a large part of the cell without mitochondria (see Fig. 2). The ellipsoid region has been shown to be very rich in succinic dehydrogenase (Wislocki and Sidman, 1954), hexokinase and malic dehydrogenase (Lowry, Roberts and Lewis, 1956; Lowry et al., 1961), all of which are required for glucose oxidation by way of the Embden-Meyerhof path and citric acid cycle. On the other hand, lactic dehydrogenase, which is required for glycolysis but not for glucose oxidation, is most abundant in the regions of the cell which have no mitochondria. This distribution agrees with the proposed separation of glucose oxidation and glycolysis in the visual cell. Other enzymes of the Embden-Meyerhof path which are required for both glycolysis and glucose oxidation were found to be abundant in the same regions of the cell that contain lactic dehydrogenase, but values for these enzymes in the ellipsoid region were not reported.

An interesting phenomenon reported by Lowry et al. (1961) is the spacial arrangement of two enzymes of the pentose phosphate path, glucose-6-phosphate dehydrogenase and 6-phosphogluconic dehydrogenase, in which the visual cells of both rabbit

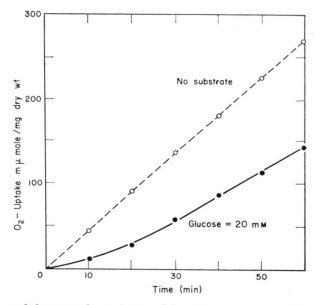

FIG. 3. Effect of glucose on the respiration of the retina of the young rabbit (5 days old).

and monkey are particularly rich. As might be expected from the fact that both of these enzymes are generally found in the soluble fraction of tissue homogenates, their activities are more or less parallel through most of the length of the visual cell, glucose-6-phosphate dehydrogenase being 3–6 times as active as 6-phosphogluconic dehydrogenase. However, in the region of the monkey visual cell nearest the outer limb there is a substantial peak in glucose-6-phosphate dehydrogenase activity but little 6-phosphogluconic dehydrogenase activity, so that the ratio of the two enzymes is over 10. (Values for these enzymes in the corresponding region of the rabbit retina were not given.) The extra glucose-6-phosphate dehydrogenase is presumably kept from diffusing by some structural element and may have some special function in visual excitation. We will return to this possibility later.

Although the conclusions reached from experiments with retinas lacking visual cells seem to agree with the histological picture, it would be desirable to obtain supporting evidence for metabolic separation of glucose oxidation and glycolysis from an examination of the metabolic properties of the normal retina. As mentioned above, tissues with a high glycolysis in the same cellular compartment as the respiratory system would be expected to display a Crabtree effect, and such an effect is in fact obtained with the young retina as seen in Fig. 3 (Cohen, 1957; Cohen and Noell, 1960). The presence of glucose in the medium inhibits oxygen uptake by 35%, which is similar to the effect reported for ascites tumors (Kun, Talalay and Williams-Ashman, 1951). In the case of the adult retina the situation is a little more complex (Fig. 4). In the presence of glucose, respiration is linear for at least 100 min. In a glucose-free medium the respiratory rate was consistently 10–12% higher for the first 40–50 min, i.e., there was a small Crabtree effect. However, after this time respiration decreased quite sharply to a slower but quite constant rate which could be maintained for a long time. It would appear from this that the initial respiration consisted of two components, one which subsided after about 50 min, and a slower more persistent one. We believe that the short-lived component of respiration is supported by carbohydrate

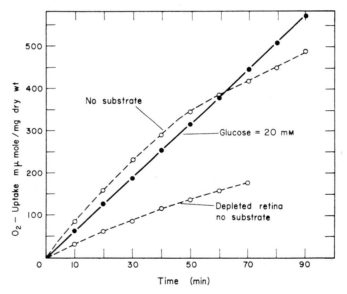

FIG. 4. Effect of glucose on the respiration of the retina of the adult rabbit. The comparison is between two retinas from a single rabbit. The depleted retina (lowest line) had been preincubated for 70 min in a 10 ml glucose-free medium, then rinsed in fresh medium and transferred to the Warburg flask.

oxidation. First, it ceases at about the same time that lactate formation ceases, i.e., when a carbohydrate store of the retina is depleted.* Second, it can be restored by the addition of glucose to the medium. The substrate of the slow, persistent respiration cannot be the lactate produced initially because retinas continue to respire at the same rate when transferred to fresh medium after 70 min incubation (the lowest line of Fig. 4). We believe this component to be supported predominantly by non-carbo-

* The glycogen content of the adult rabbit retina is about 5 times greater than that of the brain and sufficient to maintain glycolysis at a high rate for about 20 min, and then at a lower rate for about 20 min. (Cohen and Noell, 1960).

hydrate material, because it persists after the carbohydrate stores are depleted, and also because it is similar in rate to the iodoacetate-resistant respiration of the retina (Cohen and Noell, 1960). We do not mean to imply that the short-lived component can only use carbohydrate or that the persistent component can only use non-carbohydrate material, but merely that when incubated without glucose, they do use these substrates. We can now explain the small Crabtree effect and its transient nature if we assume it is confined to the persistent component. During the initial period of incubation it can be detected because the short-lived component is saturated with endogenous substrate and is not affected by the presence of added glucose in the medium; however, it is a small Crabtree effect because it involves only a minor fraction of the respiration. After the endogenous carbohydrates have been used up, however, no inhibition by glucose can be seen, because the presence of glucose stimulates the short-lived component and this masks the inhibition of the persistent component. Thus, the kinetics of respiration of the normal retina can be explained by assuming that a major component of the respiration has the following properties: it can use glucose as its principal substrate and it is exempt from the Crabtree effect (i.e., from the influence of a system of high glycolysis). A component with these properties makes its first appearance during the differentiation of the visual cell and diminishes when the visual cells are destroyed, indicating that it resides in the visual cell.

As mentioned above, histological evidence would place this component of intensive glucose oxidation in a region of the cell close to the outer segment of the rod, i.e., near the primary events of vision. This would suggest that in this highly specialized cell, the system of oxidation is assigned primarily to the amplification of the initial excitation, while glycolysis is greatly expanded in order to take over the energy support of the major part of the cell and the propagation of the amplified signal. Such specialization would take best advantage of the great energy yield of the citric acid cycle to satisfy what must be a large energy requirement for the amplification of the initial visual signal. Moreover, there seems to be a special advantage in the spatial separation of glycolysis and respiration: it would permit both activities to proceed at maximal capacity simultaneously and independently when required. From the fact that the visual cell has developed exceptional activities of these two systems, it must be assumed that it requires them at least part of the time, and spatial separation is one device to attain maximal activities. It is not possible to say at present, however, how sharp this compartmentation of systems might be.

The citric acid cycle in these cells is probably not restricted *solely* to the oxidation of glucose. There is evidence that at least glutamic acid and aspartic acid can be oxidized also* and there is no reason to assume that other substrates cannot be used. Nevertheless, what is clear is that the Embden-Meyerhof system has sufficient capacity (perhaps in conjunction with the pentose phosphate path) to feed glucose carbon into the citric acid cycle at an enormous rate,† and glucose is a very dependable energy source in most animals because its level in the blood is very well regulated.

* There are two reasons for believing glutamic acid and aspartic can be oxidized in the visual cells. First, the enzymes needed to bring these amino acids into the citric acid cycle (glutamic-oxalacetic transaminase and glutamic dehydrogenase) are concentrated in the inner limb (Lowry et al., 1956). Second, in our measurements of the oxidation of the various carbon atoms of glucose, it was found that almost 20% of the glucose carbon that entered the citric acid cycle ended up in glutamate (Cohen and Noell, 1960) and some also in aspartate (Cohen and Noell, unpublished) indicating that these compounds have access to a major site of glucose oxidation.

† The value for glucose oxidation of the adult retina given in Table I by no means represents the full capacity; it can be increased 2·7-fold by the presence of dinitrophenol in the medium, and 2·3-fold by the omission of calcium ion.

The system would seem to be specially suited to take full advantage of the citric acid cycle. It is located in a part of the cell near to the oxygen and glucose supply. Moreover, almost all of the hexokinase of the cell is confined to this region, an arrangement which would give this part of the cell first priority for glucose-6-phosphate. This arrangement might permit use of mitochondrial ATP for hexokinase, which would assure a high rate of glucose-6-phosphate formation and efficient trapping of glucose from the blood. Finally, the relatively low levels of lactic dehydrogenase in this part of the cell would minimize draining of pyruvate and reduced NAD from the system. Indeed, it might be that lactate produced in the inner regions of the cell can be used in this region of the cell and that one function of the lactic dehydrogenase in this region is to oxidize lactate rather than produce it.*

What then, might be the functional relation between glucose oxidation and the outer limb? It seems compelling to assume at least that the absorption of light by the outer limb operates some switch that either turns this glucose oxidation on (or off) or else shunts some of the energy of the system from one function to another. There are many possible ways in which this might occur. One of the simplest, which we have already suggested (Cohen and Noell, 1960) is that the outer limb might participate directly in electron transport. It is connected by solid structures (e.g., the ciliary filaments, cell membrane) to the mitochondrial cluster of the ellipsoid region, which comprises a system of enzymes capable of maintaining a high electron pressure in a small region of the cell, and it is tempting to speculate that electrons can be drawn off into the outer limb and eventually to oxygen. If, in this route, there were a gap or membrane of high resistance, and if there were a mechanism to establish a bridge across this gap when a photon is absorbed, then, upon illumination, electrons would be driven across the gap by the large redox potential drop between substrate and oxygen. If the gap were to remain closed for a finite time, the energy liberated by this electron flow would greatly exceed the energy contributed by the photon absorbed, representing a large amplification of the initial signal. This does not necessarily imply that all of the electrons involved in glucose oxidation are transported through this light-activated circuit. Only a fraction of the electrons might travel this way, generating the appropriately amplified signal. Most of the electron transport might occur by the normal mitochondrial routes, the energy obtained therefrom being used to maintain other poised systems for subsequent amplification. The most logical source of electrons for the light-activated route would seem to be NADPH, which is not directly oxidized by mitochondria. Another possible source is the NADH formed extramitochondrially during glucose oxidation (i.e., produced by glyceraldehyde-3-phosphate dehydrogenase) or during lactate oxidation, since Graymore and Towlson (1963) have reported that the activity of one of the enzymes normally required for oxidation of extramitochondrial NADH (α-glycerophosphate dehydrogenase) is very low in the retina.

There would seem to be three main questions raised by this hypothesis. (1) What is the possible nature and mechanism of the light-sensitive switch? (2) What sort of signal could be generated by the proposed electron flow, and how might it be translated into a change in membrane potential? (3) Can any evidence be adduced to support such a hypothesis other than the purely circumstantial evidence of a favourable metabolic anatomy?

As for the possible nature of the switch, one must give first consideration to rhodop-

---

* Futterman and Kinoshita (1959) have reported that the ox retina can use lactate as a substrate for respiration.

sin because it is the first material activated by light. Moreover, until the chemistry of the outer limb is better known, we have little else to include with rhodopsin. We therefore present in Fig. 5 a rather unsophisticated scheme in which rhodopsin alone is assigned the function, when suitably activated, of transporting electrons across some hypothetical gap in the circuit. There is evidence from the elegant studies of Wald, Hubbard and Kropf, and Oroshnik (see Wald, 1961) that rhodopsin, upon absorbing light, is altered in such a way that the retinylidene group is converted from the 11-*cis* isomer to the all-*trans* isomer* (see Fig. 6). According to the above hypothesis this change enables the "active rhodopsin" (possibly lumi- or meta-rhodopsin) to transport electrons. There are several ways this might occur. It has often been suggested that the isomerization of the retinylidene group might uncover an active center or produce a conformational change in the protein (see Wald, 1961). In addition, the retinene-Schiff base might be able to participate directly in electron transport when in the *trans* form but not when in the *cis* form. Provided the carbon atoms of the side chain and the atoms attached to it can lie in a single plane, the π orbitals overlap and form a molecular orbital extending from one end of the conjugated bond system to the other, through which π electrons can move. Electrons could therefore be added at one end and removed from the other by suitable donors and acceptors, respectively. Because the molecule is lipophilic it could protrude into or through a lipid barrier and carry electrons across it. In the 11-*cis* isomer, however, steric hindrance between CH_3 at C-13 and H at C-10 tends to prevent carbon atoms 10–13 from lying in a single plane and so to interrupt the molecular orbital at this point. Thus the light-induced isomerization to the *trans* form would establish a path for electron flow along the conjugated double bond system. Moreover, the change in shape from the *cis* to the *trans* form of the molecule might lengthen the retinene chain and change its position so that it penetrates the gap and comes into contact with an electron donor or acceptor. A similar mechanism for rhodopsin action has been proposed by Jahn (1963).

Such a system could generate both chemical and electrical signals, either of which might be important in visual excitation. The flow of electrons through the systems would generate chemical signals by increasing the steady state concentrations of the reduced forms of compounds in that part of the circuit following the switch, or by increasing the concentrations of oxidized intermediates preceding the switch. This can be illustrated by an example. Let us suppose that when the outer limb is activated by light it transports electrons from NADPH near the basal body of the cilium (in the ellipsoid region) to oxygen. The pentose phosphate path in the ellipsoid region should thus be stimulated. (As already mentioned, the pentose phosphate path in the retina is limited by the availability of oxidized NADP.) Moreover, since glucose-6-phosphate dehydrogenase in this region is 10 times more active than 6-phosphogluconic dehydrogenase, a high steady-state of 6-phosphogluconic acid should quickly build up. It is interesting to note that this compound is an extremely potent competitive inhibitor of phosphoglucoisomerase (Parr, 1956; Kahana, Lowry, Schulz, Passoneau and Crawford, 1960) and the possibility has been suggested that it might, in appropriate circumstances, serve to force glucose-6-phosphate into the pentose phosphate path (Kahana et al., 1960). In the enzymic environment provided by the ellipsoid region this inhibition should be especially rapid and effective. Such inhibition would assist in re-routing glucose-6-phosphate into the pentose phosphate path, thereby assuring a steady supply of NADPH for the light-activated electron transport pathway as long as

* This conversion is exergonic because the 11-*cis* form is unstable, so that the input photon need furnish only the activation energy (see Wald, 1961).

it was operative. Subsequently, if the electron flow in the outer limb were terminated,* a rapid re-establishment of the original state could occur if 6-phosphogluconate were carried by diffusion and streaming to the nearby inner region of the inner limb, where 6-phosphogluconate dehydrogenase is known to be concentrated (Lowry et al., 1961), and where other electron acceptors might provide the required NADP (e.g., pyruvate via lactic dehydrogenase). An interesting feature of this switch is that it does not cut off the supply of pyruvate to the mitochondria. After one passage of glucose-6-phosphate through the pentose phosphate path, the products (fructose-6-phosphate and phosphoglyceraldehyde) can continue on the path to pyruvate, having bypassed the blocked isomerase. The above mechanism predicts increases in the NADP/NADPH ratio and in the 6-phosphogluconate concentration in the ellipsoid region upon illumination of the retina. In addition, a decreased respiration might be expected because 6-phosphogluconate is known to inhibit mitochondrial respiration (Devlin, Barnes and Pruss, 1964) and also because the flow from glucose to pyruvate might be slower *via* 6-phosphogluconic dehydrogenase than *via* phosphoglucoisomerase. Measurements of metabolic activities and of levels of metabolites in the functioning retina thus far available fulfil some of these predictions. Low-intensity illumination decreases the reduced pyridine nucleotide level in the isolated retina (Sickel, personal communication) and decreases respiration both in isolated rods (Hanawa and Kuge, 1961) and in the intact isolated retina (Noell, this Symposium; Sickel, pers. comm.). This evidence, however, would not rule out the possibility that electrons for the light-activated path came from NADH in addition to, or instead of, NADPH, in which case the NAD/NADH ratio would be expected to increase upon illumination.

In addition to such chemical signals, an electrical signal would be generated by the above system if the proton and hydroxyl ions shown in Fig. 5 were in different

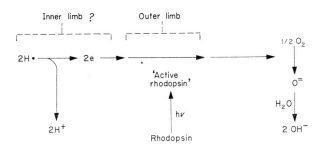

FIG. 5. Suggested role of rhodopsin in electron transport. Although the diagram indicates that electrons are removed from substrate in the inner limb and passed to oxygen in the outer limb, this direction of electron flow is not a crucial assumption of the hypothesis described in the text.

compartments. The charge separation so produced would bring about other ionic changes that might initiate the onset of further chemical processes.

Finally, let us turn to the question of evidence. Some suggestive evidence that electrons may be stripped from substrates in the inner limb and transferred to the outer

* One mechanism for termination of electron flow would be hydrolysis of metarhodopsin to retinene and opsin. This reaction appears to be the only way of terminating excitation in higher animals in bright light (Dowling and Hubbard, 1963). The retinene that is liberated by hydrolysis is reduced to retinol and migrates to the pigment epithelium. The reduction of retinene by the outer limb requires NADPH which is probably furnished by glucose-6-phosphate dehydrogenase in the outer limb (Futterman, 1963).

limb comes from histochemical studies of the localization of dehydrogenases. A number of dehydrogenases (glucose-6-phosphate dehydrogenase, NADP-linked isocitric dehydrogenase, and malic dehydrogenase) appear to be localized mainly in the outer segments when detected by tetrazolium reduction (Pearse, 1961), whereas direct measurement of two of these enzymes (glucose-6-phosphate dehydrogenase and malic dehydrogenase) in isolated fragments of the visual cell show them to be present in highest concentration in the inner segment (Lowry et al., 1956). Since the tetrazolium method does not stain the dehydrogenases *per se* but rather detects a subsequent step in electron transport, it would appear that some of the NADH and NADPH formed by these enzymes is reoxidized through the agency of the outer segment. Moreover, cytochrome oxidase has been detected histochemically in the outer limb (Akiya, 1952; Eranko, Niemi and Merenmies, 1961). Indeed, in certain respects the outer segment, with its stacks of double membranes, is not too dissimilar in appearance from a giant mitochondrion. In this regard it is of interest that the cilium-like structure of the spermatozoon of certain species has a long ribbon-like mitochondrion wrapped around it (see Lehninger, 1964), and recently, Meyer (1964) has reported that in spermatozoa of certain species of *Drosophila* these mitochondria have the form of rod-shaped, dense bodies with a regular pattern of cross striations.

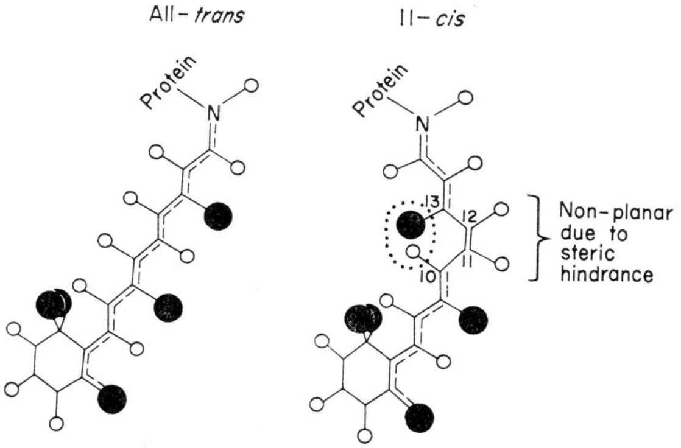

FIG. 6. Retinylidene group of rhodopsin. Open circles represent hydrogen atoms, filled circles represent methyl groups. The 11-*cis* isomer is drawn in a planar conformation in order to illustrate the steric hindrance that would occur in this conformation (modified from Dartnall, 1962).

The recent report of Falk and Fatt (1963) that the conductance of a suspension of rod outer segments increases upon illumination and returns to the original value when the rhodopsin becomes bleached would also seem to support the concept of a light-activated mechanism for electron transport. Moreover, a small receptor cell potential of no detectable latency has been recently discovered in the monkey retina by Brown and Murakami (1964). This potential is only observed with extremely intense light, such as would activate much of the rhodopsin in the visual cells. In the scheme suggested above, an intense light flash would produce a rather massive flow of electrons through the outer limb, which, because of the substantial distance involved, might be associated with a measurable potential difference. However, in its simplest form, this scheme would lead one to expect an instantaneous trans-retinal potential change opposite in polarity to the early receptor potential of Brown and Murakami (and the α-wave of the ERG).

Finally, the dependence of the electroretinogram of the isolated retina upon oxygen and glucose, which Dr. Ames has reported at this meeting, is very interesting. The fact that the effect of oxygen lack is very rapid and reversible, whereas the effect of glucose lack is not so reversible would strongly support the suggestion that oxidation is specialized for visual excitation, glycolysis for maintenance of the visual cell.

REFERENCES

Akiya, H. (1952). *Acta Soc. Ophthal. Jap.* **56**, 764.

Brown, K. T. and Murakami, M. (1964). *Nature, Lond.* **201**, 626.

Cohen, L. H. (1957). *Fedn Proc. Fedn Am. Socs. exp. Biol.* **16**, 165.

Cohen, L. H. and Noell, W. K. (1958). *Physiologist, Wash.* **1**, No. 4.

Cohen, L. H. and Noell, W. K. (1959). *Fedn Proc. Fedn Am. Socs. exp. Biol.* **18**, 28.

Cohen, L. H. and Noell, W. K. (1960). *J. Neurochem.* **5**, 253.

Dartnall, H. J. A. (1962). In *The Eye*, vol. 2, ed. by H. Davson, p. 438. Academic Press, New York.

De Robertis, E. and Franchi, C. M. (1956). *J. biophys. biochem. Cytol.* **2**, 307.

Devlin, T. W., Barnes, N. S. and Pruss, M. P. (1964.) *Biochem. Biophys. Res. Comm.* **17**, 443.

Di Pietro, D. and Weinhouse, S. (1959). *Arch. Biochem. Biophys.* **80**, 268.

Dowling, J. E. and Hubbard, R. (1963). *Nature, Lond.* **199**, 972.

Eranko, O., Niemi, M. and Merenmies, E. (1961). In *The Structure of the Eye*, ed. by G. K. Smelser, p. 159. Academic Press, New York.

Falk, G. and Fatt, P. (1963). *J. Physiol.* **167**, 36P.

Futterman, S. (1963). *J. biol. Chem.* **238**, 1145.

Futterman, S. and Kinoshita, J. H. (1959). *J. biol. Chem.* **234**, 723.

Graymore, C. N. (1959). *Br. J. Ophthal.* **43**, 34.

Graymore, C. N. (1960). *Br. J. Ophthal.* **44**, 363.

Graymore, C. N. (1964). *Nature, Lond.* **201**, 615.

Graymore, C. N. and Tansley, K. (1959). *Br. J. Ophthal.* **43**, 486.

Graymore, C. N., Tansley, K. and Kerly, M. (1959). *Biochem. J.* **72**, 459.

Graymore, C. N. and Towlson, M. (1963). *Exp. Eye Res.* **2**, 48.

Hanawa, I. and Kuge, K. (1961.) *Jap. J. Physiol.* **11**, 38.

Hubbard, R. and Kripf, A. (1958). *Ann. N.Y. Acad. Sci.* **74**, 266.

Jahn, T. L. (1963). *Vision Res.* **3**, 25.

Kahana, S. E., Lowry, O. H., Schulz, D. W., Passonneau, J. V. and Crawford, E. J. (1960). *J. biol. Chem.* **235**, 2178.

Kinoshita, J. H. (1957). *J. biol. Chem.* **228**, 247.

Kun, E. Talalay, P. and Williams-Ashman, H. G. (1951). *Cancer Res.* **11**, 855.

Lardy, H. A. and Parks, Jr., R. E. (1956). In *Enzymes: Units of Biological Structure and Function*, ed. by O. H. Gaebler, p. 584. Academic Press, New York.

Lehninger, A. L. (1964). In *The Mitochondrion*, p. 35. W. A. Benjamin, Inc. New York.

Lowry, O. H., Passonneau, J. V., Hasselberger, F. X. and Schulz, D. W. (1964). *J. biol. Chem.* **239**, 18.

Lowry, O. H., Roberts, N. R. and Lewis, G. (1956). *J. biol. Chem.* **220**, 879.

Lowry, O. H., Roberts, N. R., Schulz, D. W., Clow, J. E. and Clark, J. R. (1961). *J. biol. Chem.* **236**, 2813.

Meyer, G. F. (1964). *Z. Zellforsch. mikrosk. Anat.* **62**, 762.

Noell, W. K. (1951). *J. cell. comp. Physiol.* **37**, 283.

Noell, W. K. (1958a). *Ann. N.Y. Acad. Sci.* **74**, 337.

Noell, W. K. (1958b). *Arch. Ophthal.* **60**, 702.

Noell, W. K. (1959). *Am. J. Ophthal.* **48**, 347.

Noell, W. K. and Cohen, L. H. (1957). *Fedn Proc. Fedn Am. Socs. exp. Biol.* **16**, 95.

Parr, C. W. (1956). *Nature, Lond.* **178**, 1401.

Pearse, A. G. E. (1961). In *The Structure of the Eye*, ed. by G. K. Smelser, p. 53. Academic Press, New York.

Rose, I. A. and O'Connell, E. L. (1964). *J. biol. Chem.* **239**, 12.

Wald, G. (1961). In *The Structure of the Eye*, ed. by G. K. Smelser, p. 101. Academic Press, New York.

Warburg, O. (1927). *Biochem. Z.* **184**, 484.

Warburg, O., Posener, K. and Negelein, E. (1924). *Biochem. Z.* **152**, 309.

Wenner, C. E. and Weinhouse, S. (1956). *J. biol. Chem.* **222**, 399.

Wislocki, G. B. and Sidman, R. L. (1954). *J. comp. Neurol.* **101**, 53.

DISCUSSION

In reply to a question from DR. BRIDGES, PROFESSOR COHEN pointed out that his postulate assumed that the activated rhodopsin might act catalytically, and that during the life of this one molecule it released electron pressure across a membrane, thus creating a positive charge inside the inner segment and generating a potential. The amplification depended on the release of accumulated potential. The main problems involved defining the nature of the activated rhodopsin and determining its life. There was evidence, however, that the life of the activated metarhodopsin was considerably longer in the visual cell than when in solution.

DR. FUTTERMAN said that he felt that oxidation was a rather slow process when considered in terms of vision *per se*—one would prefer to employ it in relation to recovery processes. He felt, also, that one should be able to test such a hypothesis by looking for a cyanide insensitive respiration. PROFESSOR COHEN agreed that removal of electrons from organic substances tended to be slow, although of course, some oxidations were practically instantaneous. This might, he added, be why such a large capacity was required. By providing large quantities of intermediates such as cytochromes, rapid oxidation might well be effected. PROFESSOR COHEN agreed that he had not yet tried the effect of cyanide, although they had, in fact, examined the effect of light on respiration but had not been able to demonstrate an effect. Many others had looked for metabolic changes under such conditions, but Professor Cohen pointed out that if some *transient* form of rhodopsin were involved one might only expect an effect *during* illumination.

He also suggested that the complexity of organization in the retina would tend to obscure any specific effect on an individual element. Dr. Hanawa, working on outer segments, together with Professor Noell on the isolated frog retina, had both demonstrated a small inhibition of respiration on illumination. This *might* support the concept of a switch mechanism. When the excitatory system is open the conventional route is depressed.

In answer to DR. COLE, PROFESSOR COHEN explained that he believed a switch mechanism was necessary to explain the inhibition of respiration. It did not seem likely that the rhodopsin molecule was sufficient to drain electrons from the respiratory system, although a 'short circuit' concept had some attraction—a diversion switch seemed essential, however.

DR. ARDEN raised the objection that he felt that such a degree of amplification that could arise from the system described would not be sufficient for the needs of vision. From work he had done with Dr. Brown, the power gain of the rod appeared to be of the order of 10^{14}.

This appeared to be far too large for a single stage system, as there is no parametric amplifier that can satisfy the requirement. PROFESSOR COHEN suggested that if this applied, one might have to consider the mechanism he had described as an initial stage in the overall process of excitation.

DR. AMES said that, in view of the lack of Pasteur and Crabtree effects in the visual cells, one must assume that the inner layers exhibited these effects to a very high degree, much greater than in grey matter for example, with which one was accustomed to comparing these layers. PROFESSOR COHEN suggested the difference in magnitude of the Crabtree effect might be related to the tremendous glycolytic capacity of the inner layers. He felt that the Pasteur effect was comparable in the brain and the retina, providing that one thought in terms of both inhibition and absolute magnitude.

D

PROFESSOR COHEN closed the discussion by stressing that environment was of paramount importance. When one examined the critical requirements fulfilled by Dr. Ames, for example, in ensur-
ing a reasonable degree of electrophysiological response in the isolated retina, one had to accept
that more conventional techniques of *in vitro* study of retinal metabolism might leave much to
be desired. It could be, for example, that the loss of Pasteur and Crabtree effects in the isolated
retina reflected some degree of damage. Even so, on a comparative basis, this implies some weak-
ness of correlation that endorses the view put to the meeting. Nevertheless, he felt that studies
on appropriate media might do much to help distinguish between *in vitro capacity* and *in vivo
reality*.

Aspects of Experimental and Hereditary Retinal Degeneration*

Werner K. Noell

Department of Physiology, School of Medicine, State University of New York at Buffalo, Buffalo, N.Y., U.S.A.

This article reviews a variety of circumstances concerned in retinal degeneration, and attempts to relate these in terms of the special vulnerability of the visual cell.

In a remarkable series of essays called *"Bioenergetics"* Szent-Györgyi prefaces a speculative chapter on diseases with the following rhyme of past days, "God made the little fly. If you squash it, it will die." Ever since I learned to squash the mammalian visual cell by means of poisons (Noell, 1951, 1953a,b) I have been wondering what could be the brutal act originating from a genetic abnormality that destroys these cells in patients suffering from diseases generally referred to as "hereditary neuro-epithelial degeneration." In the following I will review retinal abnormalities in animals as they may relate to these diseases. But I might state at the outset the belief that the solution to the problem is inevitably linked to progress in biology in general. Studies on the retina provide no more perhaps than a local survey of the field in preparation for the application of principles of cell function and cell differentiation that may not yet be understood. The survey presented below is restricted to scattered areas of study in which I have personal experience. A broader view of what is known has been given by Karli (1963).

1. Manifestation of Hereditary Degeneration

To the physiologist and biochemist the degenerative visual cell diseases are presented in analogue manifestation in the mouse and the rat. The mouse disease is a sudden arrest of postnatal visual cell differentiation followed within a few days by the histological death of the cells. The final histological result is a thin retina which contains all layers except those normally occupied by the visual cells (Karli, 1952; Tansley, 1954; Noell, 1958). The outer plexiform layer which normally contains the synaptic endings of the visual cells, the eight rows of visual cell nuclei (outer nuclear layer), and the inner and outer segments have disappeared.

The most characteristic feature of this disease is its manifestation at a time when the visual cells have just differentiated to a degree which enables them to respond to light with excitation for the first time, as can be deduced from the electro-retinogram (ERG). Figure 1 compares the ERG of an afflicted mouse (C3H) with that of a control (C57 Bl). The records at the age of 11 days, that is, about 1–2 days after an electrical response to light has become recordable, are quite similar, as is also at this age the histological appearance of the retina. In this presentation I will not discuss the anatomical site and mechanisms of generation of the ERG; the ERG will be viewed merely as a convenient measure of retinal function and mainly as a null instrument for the comparison of different conditions and different ages. It should be pointed out, however, that only the first component of this response, the *a*-wave, is directly

* The research upon which this paper is based was supported by NIH grant NB-02710.

related to photoreceptor function. The subsequent components of the initial portion of the response depend upon the spread of excitation from the photoreceptor part of the cell to the proximal visual cell region and adjacent cells.

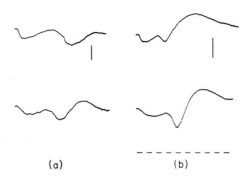

(a)   (b)

Fig. 1. ERGs of mice at the age of 11 days (a) and 12 days (b). The top tracings are from mice of the C57 Bl strain; bottom tracings are from C3H strain. The ERGs are elicited with a strong, brief xenon flash which coincides with the start of each tracing. The first (downward-negative) deflection of the record is the a-wave. Time for each tracing as indicated by dashed horizontal line, each dash representing 10 msec. Amplification for top and bottom records is as indicated by vertical lines which denote 100 μV. Note that at the age of 11 days the response of the C3H mouse (bottom) is almost as well-developed as that of the control animal (top).

The ERG changes rapidly in form and size and the minimal stimulus intensity for its elicitation decreases as outer and inner segments grow to maturity, a stage which in the mouse, rat, and rabbit is not quite reached at the age of 3 weeks. It is during the period of rapid visual cell growth, between the 12th and 18th day, that the ERG of the afflicted mouse becomes increasingly more abnormal, first of all because a-wave development is arrested (Fig. 2). The ERG becomes extinct at 20–28 days, concomitant with the death of the most disease-resistant cells near the ora serrata.

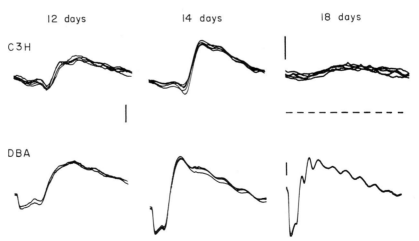

Fig. 2. ERGs at the age 12–18 days from C3H mice in comparison to ERGs of control strain (DBA). Amplification is the same for all tracings at the age of 12 and 14 days; it is twice that of the control record for the C3H mouse at 18 days. Each vertical line denotes 100 μV; each dash 10 msec.

We were unable to confirm the findings of Lucas (1958) suggesting that the hereditary degeneration in mice was still manifest, albeit retarded, under culture conditions. We performed very similar experiments using essentially the same culture technique (Trowell, 1954). The eyes were from 10-day-old animals and a large fraction of the retina survived for 5–7 days. There was no survival difference in C3H and DBA, and no histological indication that the C3H visual cells were more easily affected by the culture condition. However, neither DBA nor C3H visual cells continued with differentiation and growth. I interpret this finding as demonstrating the intimate relationship between the manifestation of the hereditary disease and visual cell differentiation. By arresting differentiation the culture condition probably also blocked the manifestation of the hereditary abnormality.

The analog disease in the rats has a later and slower manifestation (Bourne, Campbell and Tansley, 1938; Dowling and Sidman, 1962; Noell, 1963). Following an essentially normal development, the ERG at the age of 21 days is just slightly reduced but within 10 more days abnormality is clearly evident, mainly in form of a decreased and slower a-wave in response to a strong light flash. Concomitantly, here is a fall in the overall amplitude of the response, particularly to weak stimuli in the dark-adapted state. The ERG progressively decreases during subsequent weeks but it completely disappears only after 3 months provided the animals are reared in darkness (Fig. 3). The progress of the disease as demonstrated by the ERG is intimately

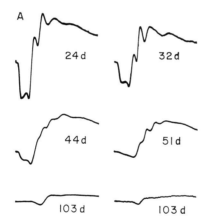

Fig. 3. ERGs of albino rats afflicted with retinal degeneration at the ages of 24–103 days. The light stimulus and recording conditions (e.g. amplification) are the same for each tracing; the animals are from the same litter reared in complete darkness. At the age of 24 days, the ERG is about the same as from a control animal, but while ERG changes little with age after 24 days, in the controls it deteriorates in the afflicted animals. The two animals tested at the age of 103 days still showed a small response originating from retinal areas near the ora serrata.

related to the appearance of histological abnormalities and to visual cell death, advancing, in the mouse, from the central region towards the periphery. The histological end result, as seen between 4–12 months, is the same as in the mouse: complete disappearance of the visual cells with preservation of the other layers (Plate 1).

2. Genetics

In both the mouse and the rat the disease is inherited as an autosomal recessive mutant. The afflicted rats studied in various laboratories all seem to derive from a strain first examined by Bourne et al. (1938). The mouse disease was discovered by Brückner (1951) and then carefully studied by Tansley (1951). There exist several inbred mouse strains with a well known history which carry the mutation; the most readily available strain is the C3H strain, of which all sub-lines so far tested (Ha, He and St) were found afflicted. The mutant gene is also carried in the prolific ICR/Ha Swiss mice, which are albinos in contrast to C3H. ICR/Ha Swiss mice are a deliberately non-inbred population. Among mice of this stock approximately 13% (59/444) were found homozygous for the mutant gene, the others accordingly, either heterozygous or homozygous for the wild-type (dominant) allele. The genetic locus in C3H and Swiss mice is the same; moreover, it can be shown that the cases of retinal mouse degeneration described in the literature from various laboratories, beginning with Brückner and Tansley, are all the expression of a mutation at the same locus (DiPaolo and Noell, 1962).

For 15 years it has been known that C3H mice (i.e., certain substrains) are markedly deficient in β-glucuronidase of major tissues such as liver, kidney and brain. The mutation responsible for the deficient production of the enzyme behaves like a simple Mendelian factor. When we tested for a possible relationship between this mutation and that responsible for visual cell degeneration, a surprisingly close linkage of these two mutations on the same chromosome was found, the two loci being only about 5 cross-over units apart (Paigen and Noell, 1961). Moreover, the two mutations showed a very similar timing of expression. As indicated by measurements of the enzyme concentration in the liver (Paigen, 1961a), animals homozygous for the recessive allele of glucuronidase production accumulated the enzyme in proportion to the postnatal increase in liver mass at the same rate as the controls up to the age of 11 days, although they started at a lower level of enzyme concentration. Subsequently, however, the increase in enzyme became rapidly slower, and after the 17th day no further enzyme accumulated. Because the liver continued to grow, enzyme concentration fell steadily until adult liver size was reached. Exactly the same pattern would be expected for the accumulation of a visual cell protein (e.g., rhodopsin) in the retina were it not for the fact that cessation of visual cell development is rapidly followed by visual cell death and lysis.

Visual cell degeneration occurs independently from the mutation for glucuronidase, and *vice versa*. However, this independent occurrence does not necessarily indicate that the functions controlled by the two loci are unrelated; on the contrary, the close linkage suggests that the two functions may have a certain biochemical system in common.

The genetic symbol for the mouse disease is rd, which stands for "retinal degeneration," the term used by Tansley in describing the disease (cf. DiPaolo and Noell, 1961). The symbol was originally proposed for the mutation as expressed in P/Jax and BDP/Jax, but it includes C3H and ICR Swiss. "Degeneration" is an appropriate noncommittal term also for similar hereditary visual cell diseases in other mammals and it is certainly a better designation than "aplasia," "abiotrophy," or "dystrophy" which are more ambitious but potentially misleading. The mouse has 20 chromosome pairs and hence at least 20 linkage groups (Gruneberg, 1943). Several of the known groups can readily be shown not to include rd, and present evidence seems to suggest that rd and g are in linkage group III (Sidman, pers. comm.). Keeler (1924) described a retinal abnormality in the mouse which attracted much attention since it showed for the first time animal retinas completely or partially devoid of visual cells. The designation of this abnormality is "rod-less," genetic symbol r. Although the strain which carried this mutation is extinct, it can be shown that r differs from rd because Keeler established linkage of r to another character ("silver") which, as we know now, segregates freely from rd (DiPaolo and Noell, 1962).

3. Rhodopsin

An established experimental procedure leading in the rat to visual cell degenera-ation concerns vitamin-A deficiency. Early research in this field (Johnson, 1943) indicated that very advanced stages of this disease were associated with the death of the visual cells, and subsequently the case was made that hereditary rod cell de-generation in man is the manifestation of a defective vitamin A metabolism (Cogan, 1950). More convincing evidence, however, of a special role of vitamin A in the main-tenance of visual cell life was obtained in experiments with vitamin A-acid supple-mentation to a vitamin A-free diet by which means the general health of the animal was maintained while visual cell death occurred after several months on the diet (Dowling and Wald, 1960). Visual cell death was preceded by a decrease in rod func-tion, as expected, and by a degeneration of the outer segments which in ultramicro-scopic appearance, interestingly, resembles that observed acutely after intravenous iodoacetate administration in rabbits (Lasansky and DeRobertis, 1959).

The ERGs recorded by Dowling (1960) during vitamin A deficiency closely resemble those of the rat during the progress of the hereditary degenerative disease. One expected to find, therefore, a decrease in rhodopsin concentration concomitant with the failure of the ERG during hereditary degeneration, or perhaps even a little earlier. The opposite, however, proved to be true, as was ascertained independently by Dowling and Sidman (1962) and Noell (1963). My results were obtained from *hooded* (pigmented) rats bred from immigrants of Dr. Graymore's line ("B-strain"). The animals were reared in dim light. Afflicted animals were mostly from a back-cross of a heterozygous F_1 generation (B × Long Evans) to the original B-strain so that they could be compared with about the same number of unaffected, heterozygous litter-mates kept in the same cage. The measurements (Noell, 1963) showed an increase in rhodopsin (extracted from the whole eye) manifest in the afflicted animals through-out the age of 20 to about 65 days. This increase became significant simultaneously with the very first start of ERG deterioration; it was greatest in percent increase from control at around the age of 28–32 days where it amounted to more than 30%, but the total content remained about the same from the age of 28–55 days. Dowling and Sidman (1962) place this increase several days earlier than Noell (1963) and they also measured a greater maximal percentage increase from their controls; the rhodopsin content of the afflicted animals was, however, virtually the same in both studies. Both studies agree, furthermore, that the rhodopsin of the afflicted animals has a normal spectrum. The same has been reported for the rhodopsin from degenerat-ing mouse retinas (Caravaggio and Bonting, 1963), where it accumulates with normal rate up to age of about 10 days and disappears simultaneously with the ERG during the 4th week of life. In the rat, rhodopsin content is still above one-fifth of normal at the age of 100 days when the ERG has almost disappeared.

These findings eliminate a localized deficiency in vitamin A or retinene availability as a primary factor in the hereditary degenerative diseases of rat and mouse. They do not, however, exclude the possibility that rhodopsin or a rhodopsin controlled reaction is an essential factor in the disease.

The rich rhodopsin content of the degenerating retina poses a problem. At the age of 50 days, for instance, a considerable fraction of the visual cell population has already disappeared in striking contrast to the high amounts of rhodopsin still present. Microscopic and electronmicroscopic evidence very strongly suggests that most of this rhodopsin is extracellular and part of a "dead" mass which occupies the space between the degenerating visual cells and the pigment epithelium (Plate 2). In osmium fixed material this very unusual tissue replacing the rods consists of membranes in form of lamellae or myelin figures which may provide a matrix for the rhodopsin (Plates 3 and 4). Incidentally, this "dead" mass can be seen with the free eye or under a lupe as an opaque layer at the outer surface of the retina when the retina is stripped off the pigment epithelium. It resembles a protein precipitate and on shaking in fluid breaks into small particles. It has a reddish color, with a brownish tint due to melanin contamination, and it bleaches through a distinct yellow. It is important to realize that this material may greatly affect determinations of dry weight or protein. In our metabolic studies as much as possible of this material was removed prior to the immersion of the retina in the flask.

There is disagreement on the origin of the membranous, rhodopsin-enriched material. Dowling and Sidman (1962), working with *albino* rats from Sorsby's stock, argue that it is most likely a product of the pigment epithelium. They seem to imply that, prior to and during rod degeneration, the pigment epithelium continuously sheds "lamellar structural constituents" together with rhodopsin until a steady state is reached and the space ordinarily occupied by the rods is filled with this extracellular tissue. I assumed that the debris derives from the degenerating rods and is mainly rod substance separated from the cell and organized into artificial membrane systems. I was led to this conclusion by the sequence of the microscopic changes which involves a gradual transition from swelling of the rods (cf. Plate 4) to the loss of a distinct structure. This view implies that the rod contains more rhodopsin prior to its disintegration than normally and that increased production of rod substance is an early manifestation of the disease. To my knowledge protein turnover studies which might provide an answer have not been performed.

4. Pigment Epithelium

The pigment epithelium of the retina and visual cells constitute a functional system as was first demonstrated 80 years ago by Kühne for rhodopsin regeneration. Their anatomical relationship is indicated by the diagram of Fig. 4 in which the fine

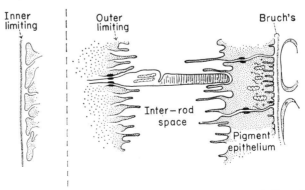

FIG. 4. Schematic drawing of relationship between rod and pigment epithelium. To the right of diagram are the choroidal capillaries. Active transport from blood to outer rod space is probably maintained by the pigment epithelium, especially by its outer, infolded surface.

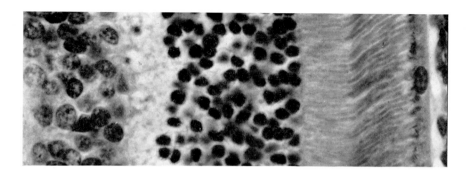

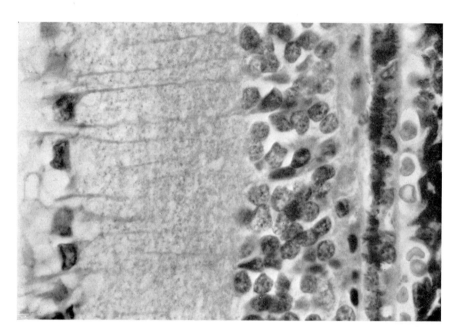

PLATE 1. Rat retina at the age of 3–4 months. Top photograph is from a control animal; bottom from afflicted animal. To the right of each picture are the choroidal capillaries. Visual cell layer of afflicted animal has almost completely disappeared; inner nuclear layer and ganglion cells are preserved. Hooded animals; hematoxylin-eosin.

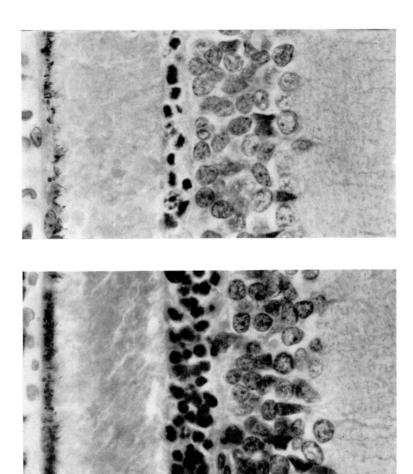

PLATE 2. Rat retina at the age of 55 (*top*) and 68 days (*bottom*). Both from afflicted animals. Note the debris in place of the rods and cones occupying the space between outer limiting membrane and pigment epithelium. The outer nuclear layer has almost disappeared in bottom photograph. Pigment epithelium seems well preserved. Hooded animals; hematoxylin-eosin.

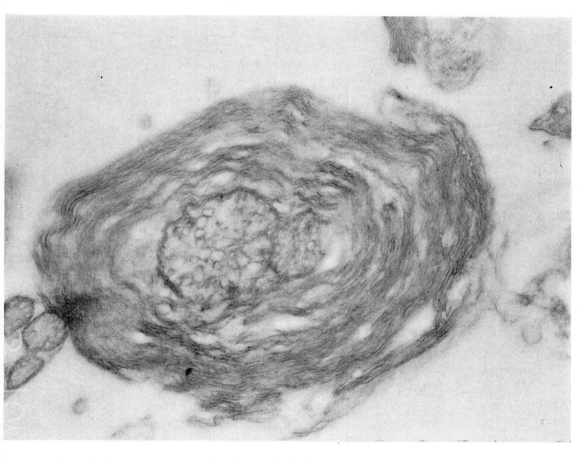

PLATE 3. Electronmicrograph of "rod" space during debris phase. Illustrated is a "myelin" figure between outer limiting membrane and pigment epithelium. Hooded rat at the age of 41 days. Osmium ($\times$ 10,000). (From unpublished material obtained by DeRobertis, Lasansky and Noell in 1961.)

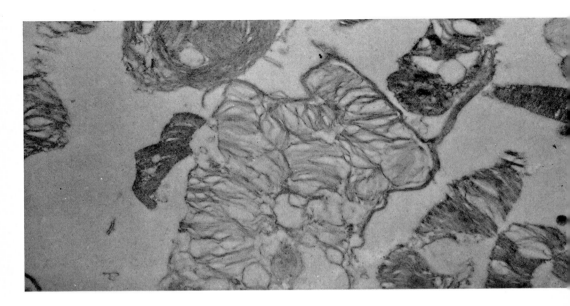

PLATE 4. Electronmicrograph of degenerating rods. Hooded rat; 38 days old. Note the swollen, deteriorating rod in center of figure. Osmium (×6000). (From DeRobertis, Lasansky and Noell, unpublished.)

apical processes of the pigment epithelium are shown to extend far into the (narrow) spaces between the outer segments which they indeed enclose. There is much evidence that the integrity of visual cell function and structure, especially for long range maintenance, depends upon the pigment epithelium but, conversely, pigment epithelial function is to a certain degree dependent upon the visual cells. Electrophysiologically, this relationship is indicated by certain slow waves of the ERG that are generated by the pigment epithelium in response to the stimulation of the visual cells by light. The pigment epithelium is also the site of a major fraction of the transretinal ohmic resistance and capacitance and it seems to generate most of the steady d.c. potential across the eye as an electrical manifestation of active ion transport (cf. Noell, 1963). This transport seems specifically sensitive to azide since intravenous injection produces a rapid rise of the transocular potential difference which, within limits, is proportional to the instantaneous concentration of azide in the choroidal blood (Noell, Crapper and Paganelli, 1964).

The electrical reaction to azide is a means of ascertaining the functional state of the pigment epithelium after the degeneration of the visual cells when light-induced reactions can no longer be obtained. In the rat with hereditary retinal degeneration azide responsiveness was maintained at the age of 120 days (Fig. 5) and at least up

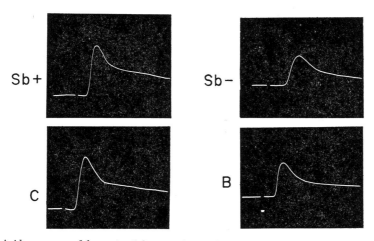

FIG. 5. Azide response of d.c. potential across the eye in rats. At the interruption of each line near its start azide solution (0·2 ml, 10^{-3}M) is injected into tail vein; 3–5 sec later the d.c. potential rises several mV, reaches a peak and slowly returns to base line. *Left column:* "normal" rats; *right column:* afflicted rats. Top records are from (hooded) littermates at the age of 132 days; the left record is from a heterozygous, "normal" rat (Sb+), the right record is from a homozygous, "abnormal" animal (Sb −) which does not show a response to light. *Bottom:* left record (C) is from a (normal) Long Evans rat; right record (B) is from an afflicted rat of the "B" strain; both about 4 months old. Note that response to azide is preserved, though lower in amplitude, despite virtually complete degeneration of the visual cells.

to the age of 1 year. The reaction was definitely reduced in magnitude, the more so the older the rat, and to some greater extent in afflicted albino rats of our breeds than in hooded animals. The question of a primary or secondary involvement of the pigment epithelium in hereditary degeneration has plagued the literature but nothing definite can be said. Unquestionably, the visual cells die while the pigment epithelium survives, though altered in functional capacity, for at least several months. Both cell populations may be affected by the same mutation as may be all other cells of the retina or, for that matter, of the body; we simply do not know.

By means of the electrical reactions it is possible to decide quite clearly whether or not a certain experimental procedure affects first the pigment epithelium or the visual cells. A good example is the effect of sodium iodate which when administered intravenously produces within hours or days a degeneration of the visual cells which has been likened, erroneously I feel, to typical hereditary visual cell degeneration (Sorsby, 1941). Figure 6 illustrates that the first effect of the poison in the rabbit is upon transretinal potential changes which previously (Noell, 1953b) were suggested to depend on the integrity of the pigment epithelium. These are certain slow waves (e.g. the c-wave) in response to light stimulation, and the electrical reaction to intravenous or intra-arterial sodium azide. Histology agrees with this assumption in that the most outstanding effect of iodate is not the death of the visual cells but the disintegration of the pigment epithelium in association with the degeneration of outer and inner segments.

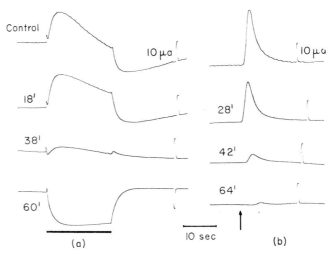

Fig. 6. Effect of iodate in rabbit on slow ERG waves (a) and the response to azide (b). The animal is in urethane anesthesia; anterior part of eye bulb is replaced by a fluid filled cylinder (cf. Noell, 1963). Recorded is the transretinal current with voltage clamped at zero (so-called "short-circuit" current) At the left, eye is illuminated steadily for 20 sec as indicated by heavy bottom line; the large, upward response following "on" is the c-wave which disappears within 1 hr (60′) following intravenous injection of sodium iodate (at 0 time). The response to azide tested during the intervals between light stimuli, diminishes simultaneously with c-wave. The large negative (downward) wave replacing the c-wave probably is a visual cell potential whereas c-wave seems to depend upon the integrity of pigment epithelium.

As one would expect from the close relationship between pigment epithelium and visual cells, many poisons or procedures which specifically affect the one population also seem to have the potential of directly interfering with the viability of the other. The decision as to direct or indirect effect is generally impossible and all that can be done is to determine the time sequence of the changes. In relation to the iodate effect, it may be worthy of note that α-tocopherol (Babel and Ziv, 1956) and cysteine (Sorsby and Harding, 1960) seem to provide some protection.

5. Glucose Metabolism

The selectiveness of the degeneration of the visual cells on the basis of a single gene mutation can be viewed as the expression of a particular vulnerability of the visual cell to a specific disturbance of cellular or enzymatic activities. Indeed the visual cell takes a unique position among the retinal cell populations as regards the effectiveness of certain poisons that interfere with specific metabolic activities. The action of iodoacetate (IAA) is perhaps the most outstanding example. Within minutes after intravenous injection of IAA, visual cell function is completely lost; and if the poison is given in a dose higher than is necessary for effects upon visual cell excitation (ERG) the visual cells show pyknosis and other manifestations of visual cell death within 12–14 hr. The ultimate histological result after lysis of the cells is the same as in hereditary degeneration, i.e., the virtually complete disappearance of the visual cell layers with little or no effect upon any other layer.

Three other phenomena made the IAA effect an intriguing analog of the hereditary disease: (1) in monkey retinas IAA destroyed the rod cell population while the cone cells survived so that foveal visual capacities were preserved as in typical retinitis pigmentosa; (2) the effectiveness of IAA in producing visual cell death in the adult animal was according to the anatomical pattern of early post-natal visual cell differentiation, i.e., as the dosage was increased, cell death progressed towards the periphery; (3) the IAA effectiveness was age dependent. The visual cell vulnerability became evident first in rabbits at the age of 20 days and then increased up to the age of several months. In addition, ERG studies of the acute effects of IAA and anoxia revealed that the metabolic organization of the rod cells differs among mammalian species, most notably between the rabbit and mammals such as cat and monkey (Noell, 1951). We know now that the rat falls into the cat and monkey category, whereas the guinea pig behaves like the rabbit as regards the earliest change in the form of the ERG. Rabbit and guinea pig differ from the other mammals in that they do not possess an intraretinal capillary network; their retinal nutrition depends exclusively upon supply by the choroidal capillaries. Apparently, in relation to this dependency upon supply by the choroidal blood vessels, the most acutely susceptible visual cell region is located more proximal to the synaptic ending than in the other species. Similar species differences are apparent in the retinal distribution of TPN- and DPN-dependent enzymes of glycolysis and respiration (Lowry, Roberts and Lewis, 1956), and these differences are also evident ultra-microscopically with respect to the presence or absence of a mitochondrion in a synaptic spherule of the visual cell.

As regards the primary action of IAA a good case can be made that this action is upon triose phosphate dehydrogenase, and that the loss of visual cell function results from the depression of metabolic energy production to critical levels. It is less clear whether the relative effectiveness of iodoacetate upon the visual cells is the expression of a special dependency of the visual cells upon ATP produced by the Embden-Mayerhof pathway or upon glucose as the main substrate of non-oxidative and oxidative (Krebs cycle) activities. The first possibility is strongly favored on the basis of physiological evidence (ERG effects) especially by a comparison of the action of iodoacetate and oxygen withdrawal (Noell, 1951), whereas the second possibility is suggested by *in vitro* measurements (Noell, 1959). *In vitro* glucose oxidation of the adult rabbit retina accounts for the major portion of respiration and only about 30% of the oxygen uptake is due to the oxidation of non-carbohydrate substrates (Cohen and Noell, 1960). Hence, iodoacetate, at concentrations which depress aerobic and anaerobic lactic acid production by more than 40% also reduces respiratory rate, apparently because the utilization of endogenous substrate for oxidation is limited and can compensate for no more than a 20% reduction in glucose oxidation (Table I).

However, the *in vivo* effects of iodoacetate occur when lactic acid production is inhibited probably by no more than 50%. It is, of course, possible that glycolysis supplies some metabolic intermediate essential for the maintenance of visual cell life or perhaps even visual cell excitation.

TABLE I

In vitro *effects of IAA, added to medium*

IAA M	Anaerobic lactic acid	Aerobic lactic acid	Glucose oxidation	O_2 consumption	Oxidation of endogenous carbon sources
			Adult retina		
1×10^{-5}	85	92	92	100	117
5×10^{-5}	58	62	79	95	130
1×10^{-4}	33	32	50	75	130
2×10^{-4}	12	18	32	59	120
1×10^{-3}	<2	5	6	39	111
			Young retina		
2×10^{-3}	7	10	12	90	123

Metabolic activities are expressed as per cent of control measurements

TABLE II

In vitro *activities of degenerating rat retinas (ss)*
in comparison to "normal" retinas (S)

Age	Strain	CO_2 production from [U-^{14}C]glucose ("glucose oxidation")	Aerobic lactic acid	Anaerobic lactic acid
22–28 days	ss	440 (4)	850 (7)	1380 (5)
	S	450 (4)	790 (4)	1600 (4)
34–40 days	ss	395 (7)	520 (8)	1880 (14)
	S	440 (12)	860 (12)	2050 (12)
50–58 days	ss	380 (12)	460 (6)	2030 (4)
	S	420 (5)	850 (4)	2070 (4)
70–74 days	ss	400 (6)	550 (6)	1830 (7)
	S	370 (6)	820 (6)	2070 (13)

All values are in mμmoles/mg dry wt/hr. Number of experiments from which average was computed as indicated in parenthesis.

The effects of iodoacetate upon the visual cells stimulated the measurement of metabolic activities of retinas prior to and during the manifestation of hereditary degeneration by Graymore, Tansley and Kerly (1959), Walters (1960), Graymore (1960) and Brotherton (1962). They studied the afflicted rat strain and all agree that glycolysis is reduced but, as Graymore (1964) puts it, "It is difficult to relate this with any degree of accuracy to the time of onset of the histological changes." My measurements on the rat fully support this view. They were performed according to techniques developed by Professor L. Cohen, using Krebs-Ringer-glucose-phosphate medium containing calcium, and an enzymatic assay for lactic acid determinations (Cohen and Noell, 1960). The animals were of the hooded type reared in dim light. Controls were either heterozygous litter mates or from a heterozygous F_1 generation. The retinas were dissected free in saline solution with visual inspection through a stereoscopic lupe. Dead tissue or non-retinal tissue was carefully separated from the retina. A single Warburg flask contained one retina in 0·84 ml solution, in air or nitrogen. Incubation for measurement was for 70 min. Results were related to mg dry weight. Mean data of these measurements are presented in Table II. The animals were clearly different in their ability to produce lactic acid aerobically, this difference becoming apparent at 4 weeks of age. For earlier stages of the disease a great number of experiments would be required, such as were performed by the aforementioned authors, to demonstrate any difference that might exist under the conditions of my experiments. It is evident from the results shown in Fig. 2 that no difference can be shown, even for advanced stages of the disease, in anaerobic lactic acid formation and in the production of CO_2 from uniformly labeled [^{14}C]glucose. The main difference, therefore, is in the magnitude of the Pasteur effect.

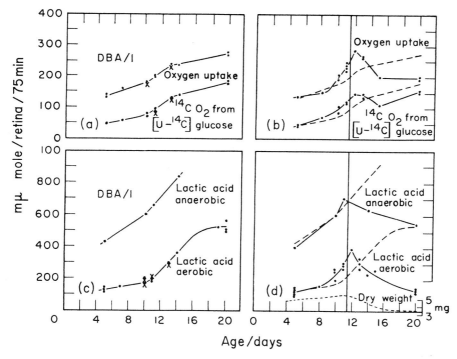

Fig. 7. Metabolic activities measured *in vitro* with retinas from normal control strain (DBA/1) (a) and (c); and from rd strains (C3H); or afflicted Swiss (b) and (d). The vertical line in (b) and (d) marks the 11 1/2 day of age at which time visual cell pyknosis becomes first evident. The dashed lines refer to the DBA data; heavy lines and dots ((b) and (d)) represent rd (e.g. C3H) data.

From Cohen's studies (1957) and Lowry's data (1956) on enzyme distribution in rabbit and monkey retina a control of glycolysis by respiration may be expected relatively more for the inner retinal layers than for the visual cells. There are then two interpretations possible for the low aerobic glycolysis of the afflicted rats. One is that the bulk of the measured metabolic activities after the age of 3 weeks resides within the inner layers and that these layers determine the activity pattern, the other that the degenerating visual cells shift in their metabolic pattern to one more typical for the immature visual cells than for the adult or, in other words, that they undergo a kind of metabolic de-differentiation.

Similar and more extensive experiments were performed on mice. Experimental conditions were essentially the same as in the study of the rat retina except that 4 whole retinas were incubated per Warburg flask for most ages. The results shown in Fig. 7 are expressed per 1 retina for several reasons: (a) it proved easy to dissect the whole mouse tissue without any apparent loss in both the control and afflicted strains; (b) dry weight of the flask contents for any age or any strain showed greater variations than the measured activities, suggesting that weight was the least accurately measured quantity; (c) total activities, (activities per whole retina) relate better to histological changes than do specific activities. The control strain was DBA/1, and its activities show the characteristic rapid increases between the age of 9–20 days, coinciding with the development of the ERG from earliest appearance to mature size. As in the rabbit (Cohen and Noell, 1960), glucose oxidation increased more than oxygen uptake, and aerobic lactic acid formation more than anaerobic.

There were no significant differences between C3H retinas and those of controls up to the age of about 8 days. For the next 4 days, however, C3H activities, with the exception of anaerobic lactic acid production, exceeded control values. This increase from normal became more evident from day-to-day and reached peak values at about 12 days. Thereafter, all activities decreased, most sharply and extensively aerobic lactic acid production. This phase of the metabolic changes almost exactly coincided with the first appearance of visual cell death and its progress over the population. However, specific activities computed on the basis of average dry weight indicate a decrease only for aerobic glycolysis; specific oxygen uptake, glucose oxidation and anaerobic glycolysis at 15–20 days differ little between C3H and DBA.

The increased metabolic activities prior to cell death suggest a failure of the cell to restrain oxidation and aerobic glycolysis. Ultra-structural changes (DeRobertis and Lasansky, 1961) point in the same direction in that the inner segments display excessive amounts of vesicles and granules and pathological formation of lamellar membranes.

The contribution of the various carbon atoms of exogenous glucose to the CO_2 produced was measured in mice using the same techniques as reported by Cohen and Noell (1960). The data (Table III) for the age of 5 days are identical for C3H and DBA, including the oxidation of C–1 when unlabeled pyruvate is added, and with or without iodoacetate, in order to examine the operation of the pentose phosphate pathway. The pattern of these activities is not significantly different from the one analyzed for the young rabbit retina (Cohen and Noell, 1960).

At the age of 10 days most activities of the C3H retina differ from the controls but a close examination of these data with others obtained from slightly older animals fails to reveal a specific abnormality. The higher values recorded for C3H are obtained with about the same pattern of distribution in controls only 1–3 days older. As shown above, metabolic activities rapidly increase at this age and, in fact, change from one day to the other in a very consistent manner which perhaps illustrates the fact that the animals are from well established inbred lines.

A distinctly different pattern, however, is evident at the age of 20 days when the visual cell population is reduced to a small number (Table III). While total activities in normal medium are lower throughout, pyruvate addition to the medium fails to stimulate C–1 oxidation preferentially. However, the addition to the medium of an artificial electron acceptor, phenazine methosulfate (2×10^{-4}M) which in rabbit retina and ascites cells increases the oxidation of C–1 many times over that observed with pyruvate, stimulates this activity in afflicted and non-afflicted animals to about the same extent. Incubation with phenazine was for 20 min instead of the usual 75 min, but results are expressed as for the other measurements. Different conditions were tested in relation to these findings and the results compared (Table IV) in terms

TABLE III

Pattern of glucose oxidation in C3H and DBA or equivalent mice

Age	Strain	[U-^{14}C]	[6-^{14}C]	[1-^{14}C]	[1-^{14}C] Pyruvate added	[1-^{14}C] Pyruvate added $+2 \times 10^{-4}$ IAA	[1-^{14}C] Phenazine methosulfate added
5 days	C3H	50	2·3	4·2	5·8	7·0	
	DBA	49	2·3	4·5	5·4	7·3	
10 days	C3H	92	7·5	8·7	11·0	7·4	
	DBA	72	3·4	5·9	7·5	7·5	
20 days	C3H	154	15	19	9·4	1·7	153
	DBA	195	21	25	21·5	7·3	164

Aerobic: Krebs-Ringer-phosphate with 16 mM glucose. Values are expressed in mμmoles ^{14}CO$_2$ produced per retina during 75 min of incubation from glucose labeled as indicated.

TABLE IV

Preferential 1–^{14}C oxidation expressed as the difference (mμmoles)
from 1–^{14}C and 6–^{14}C labeled glucose

Strain	Aerobic condition (60% O$_2$)	Aerobic pyruvate added	Anaerobic pyruvate added	Aerobic pyruvate added $+10^{-4}$M IAA	Aerobic $+2 \times 10^{-4}$M phenazine methosulfate
C3H	4·1	5·4	5·5	1·3	147
DBA	4·3	13	15	4·4	153

Same or similar experiments as in Table III.
Mice at the age of 20 days.

of preferential C–1 oxidation, i.e., C–6 oxidation subtracted from C–1 oxidation, both these being measured simultaneously on the same litter in different flasks. No difference between the strains exists for incubation in glucose medium equilibrated with oxygen enriched air (60% O$_2$). Likewise, there is no difference for the equivalent anaerobic conditions (not shown) for which preferential C–1 oxidation is reduced to about one-third. However, while pyruvate (10 mM) stimulates C–1 oxidation by a factor of 3–4 in DBA, it does so only by 20% in C3H for both the aerobic and anaerobic conditions. This difference is also evident in the presence of iodoacetate (IAA) suggesting that the availability of glucose-6-phosphate is limiting to the same degree in both strains when glycolysis is blocked. In view of the equally high rates of decarboxylation in the presence of phenazine methosulfate, a lack in substrate or a depression in activity of the enzymes of the oxidative shunt cannot be the basis for the absence of the response to pyruvate. It rather seems as if pyruvate is not a suitable electron acceptor in the C3H retina at the age of 20 days.

Graymore (1964) showed that the retinal isoenzyme fraction 5 of lactic dehydrogenase varies in the rat with age. Compared to the other fractions its activity was markedly enhanced in the young immature retina of normal animals in contrast to the pattern in the adults. In young rats of the afflicted strain, fraction patterns resembled that of the normal adult; in fact, a slight decrease was evident instead of the normal increase. Adult afflicted rats showed this decrease more conspicuously. Graymore's data suggest that fraction 5 of LDH plays a role in retinal differentiation, and he speculates that this fraction may control oxidative shunt activity. The basis of the argument is the finding in rabbits (Cohen and Noell, 1960), which the results of Table IV on mice confirm, that the operation of the pentose phosphate path is normally much restricted by the availability of electron acceptors for TPN regeneration, and that in vitro addition of pyruvate may remove some of this restriction by coupling TPNH oxidation to lactate formation from added pyruvate.

It is possible to explain the absence of a pyruvate response in the 20-day-old rd retina by assuming a deficiency in TPNH utilization as a co-factor in the conversion of pyruvate to lactate as suggested by Graymore's data on the rat. One must consider, however, that this deficiency may be the expression of a normal difference in activities between the inner retinal layers of the mouse and the visual cells which becomes evident after visual cell death. The same interpretation may apply to the low aerobic production of lactic acid; i.e., the manifestation of a greater Pasteur effect than in the controls.

Conventional in vitro measurements of retinal glycolysis, respiration and glucose oxidation do not produce simple answers mainly for two reasons: (1) the retina is a heterogenous tissue and the participation of the various populations in the measured activities cannot be resolved; (2) the condition of measurement imposes a severe stress upon the tissue by the use of artificial medium, the trauma of shaking and the very fact that the retina is separated from its natural relationship to other parts of the eye. An unspecified abnormality, therefore, is added to whatever abnormality exists in vivo and the response to the induced abnormality probably varies depending on the in vivo state of the tissue. It is quite clear, for instance, that in vitro rates of respiration are considerably higher than in vivo, more so in bicarbonate than in phosphate buffer (Cohen and Noell, 1960).

In view of these considerations and the data at hand, it is probably fair to state that, on the basis of these measurements, no good case can be made for or against a primary deficiency in energy yielding reactions of glucose metabolism in hereditary degeneration. The question then is whether any case can be made at all. At the present this can be answered only intuitively, and my intuition is that none exists. Unquestionably, however, the ultimate event in the chain of reactions by which the mutation causes cell death will involve metabolic energy production, and the depression of this activity may well be the immediate cause of cell death. This will become self-evident in the next part of our discussion.

6. Visual Cell Vulnerability

In addition to iodoacetate there are several experimental procedures, reviewed in the following, which produce visual cell death acutely and in approximately as selective a manner as iodoacetate, the hereditary condition or vitamin A deficiency.

All these effects when viewed together lead to the conclusion that the vulnerability of the visual cells to iodoacetate is not simply the manifestation of an unusual dependency upon glycolysis but, in addition, the expression of some other peculiarity which makes the visual cells more vulnerable than the other retinal cells. The only exception which is perhaps very significant is the suppression of respiration by the lack or absence of oxygen to which the visual cells are more resistant than bipolar cells and ganglion cells; in fact, resistance to the irreversible effect of anoxia is very high for the retina as a whole in comparison to brain and other organs.

X-Irradiation

X-Irradiation, like IAA, affects the rod cells much more than the cone cells and any other retinal cell populations. Characteristic of its action is the sudden disappearance of visual cell function as measured by the ERG in rabbits when a critical dose (approximately 4–5000 rads) has been attained (Noell, 1962a). This effect occurs within no more than a few minutes after the critical dose level has been reached. The effect is irreversible, i.e., histological manifestations of visual cell death develop invariably within a few hours or at least 1 day after a change in the ERG. This close relationship between the destruction of a vital visual cell function and effects upon the excitatory processes (observed by means of the ERG) is not the result of a particular type of X-irradiation because we have varied dose rate, dose schedule, and the quality of irradiation (80–2000 KVP) in extensive experiments without finding an exception to this relationship. Doses of X-irradiation which are no more than 10% lower than those producing acute visual cell death may impair specifically the outer segment, leading to a degeneration similar to the one observed after iodate administration; but this histological effect becomes apparent with delay and is best observed with dose fractionation over several weeks.

TABLE V

Effects of X-irradiation on in vitro activities

Dose* (rads)	ERG† b-wave	O$_2$-uptake	Glucose oxidation	Lactic acid aerobic	Lactic acid anaerobic
			mμmoles/dry wt/hr		
0	—	470 (16)	310 (12)	644 (16)	960 (4)
			% change from control		
1300	—	−6 (2)	0 (2)	+5 (2)	—
2600	±5 (4)	−8 (4)	−6 (4)	−2 (4)	—
3400	+12 (6)	−3 (6)	−11 (6)	−3 (6)	—
4200	−55 (2)	−32 (2)	−51 (2)	+1 (2)	—
5000	−82 (10)	−52 (6)	−71 (5)	−2 (6)	−24 (4)
6000	−96 (4)	−57 (4)	−74 (4)	−5 (4)	—

* Medium retinal dose.
† Measured 20 min after irradiation. Number of experiments is given in parenthesis.
Measured for 1 hr starting 1/2 hr after irradiation.

The acute effects of X-irradiation upon visual cell viability and ERG were associated closely with metabolic changes. This was shown in experiments in which the retina was removed 25 min after the start of 2000 KVP irradiation of the eye of rabbits. The retinas were immediately incubated in Warburg flasks (glucose-Krebs-Ringer-phosphate) and metabolic activities measured during the following hour. Dose rate of irradiation was constant (300 rads/min) and total dose was varied by

E

changing the duration of exposure between 4 and 20 min. The ERG in response to 0·5 sec flashes of light was recorded continuously during exposure and thereafter, and the last measurement was taken just prior to eye removal. Table V lists the results. Clearly, doses below the critical level of effectiveness upon the ERG (i.e., up to about 3800 rads) did not alter metabolic activities in comparison to the control. However, when the dose was sufficient to affect the ERG, and hence destroyed visual cell viability, metabolic activities were decreased in proportion to the ERG effect. This decrease did not occur with respect to aerobic or anaerobic lactic acid formation; it was restricted clearly to mitochondrial activities. On the basis of arguments which have been given elsewhere (Noell, 1962a), it is very difficult to relate these mito- chondrial activity changes to those of the ERG in terms of a cause-and-effect rela- tionship. It rather seems as if X-irradiation affects the visual cell diffusely and that at the critical dose level a "protective" mechanism has been destroyed to the extent that all membrane-bound functions of the visual cell disappear. If the X-ray dose is below the critical level, this "protective" mechanism recovers with an initial rate constant of about 2 hr, as expressed by the rate of recovery of the latent X-ray effect tested by a second exposure at varying times following exposure to a just ineffective dose.

Oxygen poisoning

Oxygen at a pressure of several atmospheres has long been known to be lethal, producing death either by CNS failure (preceded by convulsions) or by pulmonary damage. Gerschman, Gilbert, Nye, Dwyer and Fenn (1962) suggested that these effects of oxygen result from the formation of free radicals in the metabolizing tissue, and by experiments with protective agents such as those used against X-irradiation they were able to support this hypothesis. Their hypothesis stimulated our studies of several years ago (Noell, 1962b). It was found that O_2 pressure above 0·5 atm. produces reduction and disappearance of the rabbit's ERG after an accumulated period of time which was inversely related to oxygen pressure. This ERG effect was best studied at O_2 pressures above 3 atm. At these pressures the decline of the ERG started suddenly, and once it started progressed steadily to complete disappearance (Fig. 8) in a manner which was typical also for the X-irradiation effect (Fig. 9). Both

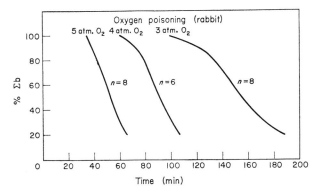

FIG. 8. Time course of the effect of high O_2 pressures upon ERG in % of control amplitude of b-wave (Eb). The lines represent the average ERG change in n experiments. Abcissa: time from start of exposure to indicated O_2 pressure. During exposure to 3 atm. of oxygen, for instance, the ERG remained un- changed for about 100 min; it then fell steadily in amplitude to reach the 50% level on the average at 155 min after the start of exposure. The b-wave was 20% of control size at 180 min. The ERG decline at various pressures is the manifestation of the accumulative action of oxygen.

effects, hence, displayed the same accumulative mode of action suggesting a similarity in their mechanism of action.

In order to prove that the ERG effect of high O_2 pressures was truly the result of an increased O_2 pressure within the retinal tissue, the intraocular pressure of one eye of rabbits was kept steadily increased (e.g., at 50 mmHg) in order to reduce in this

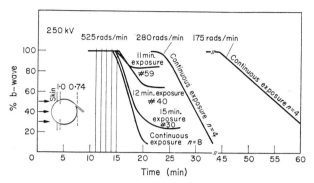

FIG. 9. The accumulative action of X-irradiation measured by the ERG. Average ERG declines are drawn from n experiments as in Fig. 8. Abcissa: time from start of irradiation; 250 kV at different dose rates. Dose (e.g., 525 rads/min) is expressed as the median dose to which the retinal cells are exposed when the X-ray beam enters the eye anteriorly (e.g., through cornea). The retinal cells near the cornea are exposed to a greater dose than those located more posteriorly depending upon radiation quality. With 250 kV radiation, exposure of posterior pole cells is 74% that of the anterior cells (see insert to left of figure). Irradiation is continuous through the ERG decline except for the 3 experiments individually drawn in which exposure to 525 rads/min was terminated after 11 min (exp. #59), 12 min (exp. #40) and 15 min (exp. #30). In these experiments, therefore, the ERG decline occurred after cessation of X-irradiation thus providing a measure of the critical dose required to affect the ERG. The incomplete fall of the ERG in these cases is the manifestation of the fact that only the anterior parts of the retina were sufficiently exposed when exposure time was shortened.

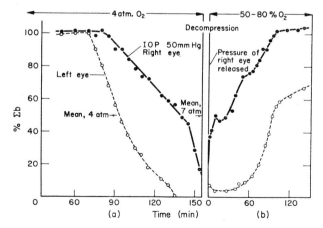

FIG. 10. ERG decline during exposure to 4 atm. O_2 and recovery following decompression to ambient pressure. Oxygen pressure during recovery was (for certain reasons) slightly above normal (50–80%) instead of the normal 20%. The ERG is measured from both eyes; the IOP of right eye is increased throughout exposure to high O_2 to 50 mmHg by the application of a steady pressure through a cannula in anterior chamber; the left eye serves as control. As shown, the ERG of right eye is markedly less affected than control eye by the increased inspiratory O_2 pressure because the retinal O_2 pressure of right eye is prevented from reaching the same light level as in left retina. Recovery from effect of O_2 also is faster in right eye.

eye ocular circulation and O_2 pressure in comparison to the other eye during O_2 exposure. As shown in Fig. 10 the impairment of ocular circulation indeed delayed the appearance of an ERG effect as would be predicted for a direct effect of O_2 upon the retina.

Metabolic effects of O_2 poisoning and X-irradiation also were similar. Because of the rapidly lethal action of O_2 at high pressures, metabolic activities had to be measured on isolated retinas (from DBA mice) which were exposed to a high O_2 pressure while incubated in flasks. During a 1 hr exposure to 6 atm. of oxygen, glucose oxidation was only 30% that of the controls. The percentage of inhibition was less in relation to exposures shorter than 1 hr. As in the X-ray experiments, there was no reduction in lactic acid formation.

As was described for X-irradiation and other procedures, O_2 poisoning produced selective visual cell death when the animals were exposed to pressures which they were capable of surviving for at least 12 hr. Visual cell death even occurred consistently at 1 atm. of O_2 with exposure times of about 40 hr. The lowest effective O_2 pressure was about 6/10 atm. In contrast to X-irradiation, the ERG effect was not irreversible and in order to produce visual cell death at 1 atm. pressure, the animals had to be exposed for several hours beyond the start of an ERG change; otherwise complete recovery occurred. Furthermore, the earliest signs of an ERG effect at several atm. O_2 were not the same as during X-irradiation and indicated that the effect of O_2 is initially more localized in the visual cell than that of X-irradiation.

It should be pointed out that in relation to our main theme, visual cell death from O_2 poisoning showed the same anatomical location and progress as the effect of iodoacetate; cells near the center of the retina were most susceptible and those at the ora serrata the least. Thus, despite the fact that the two agents differ most probably in their primary mechanism of action, they destroyed the visual cell population according to the same distribution of vulnerability. Furthermore, the effectiveness of O_2 poisoning depended upon the state of visual cell development or maturity in a similar manner as the effectiveness of iodoacetate.

Light induced damage

Since the turn of the century it has been known that visible light may be injurious to plant and animal cells, especially in the presence of artificial photosensitizing substances. Curiously, effects of this kind have never been considered in relation to the retina although they are well recognized in dermatology. Recent observations, however, suggest that excessive light has the potential of adversely affecting the visual cells.

Dowling and Sidman (1962) first reported that the hereditary disease in rats progresses strikingly faster in animals reared in light instead of in the dark. We attempted to quantitate this effect by exposing the rats at various stages of the disease to strong light for varying periods of time. A typical result is shown in Fig. 11.

Hooded (eye pigmented) rats of the afflicted strain were kept in the dark throughout life until the age of 35 days, at which time the disease was only moderately advanced and the ERG moderately abnormal. Half of the litter was then exposed to a light environment of 30-ft candles for 24 hr (i.e., for the 36th day after birth) and thereafter replaced in the dark. The ERGs recorded during the subsequent weeks clearly were lower and more affected in those animals that had been exposed to light (E) than in the control littermates (D). Interestingly, the disease progressed in the exposed animals as if in comparison to the controls, the 1-day-exposure had advanced the "functional age" of the visual cells by about 30 days. The ERG recorded at the age of 60 days, for instance, was as low as usually observed at about the age of 90 days. Histological examination led to the same conclusion.

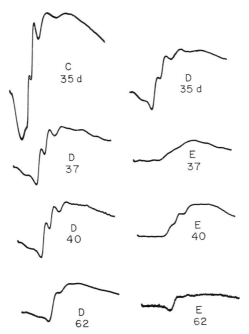

FIG. 11. Effect of 24 hr exposure to light on progress of retinal degeneration in rats. ERGs of albino rats; C— normal control rat (Sprague-Dowley strain) at age of 35 days; the other ERGs are from a litter of afflicted, albino rats reared in darkness. At the age of 36 days, one-half of the litter was exposed to bright light for 24 hr and then again maintained in darkness. *Left column:* Typical ERGs of rats (D) maintained constantly in darkness; *right column:* typical ERGs of animals (E) which were exposed to light at the age of 36 days. Note that at the age of 62 days, retinal degeneration is much more advanced in the E— than in the D animals; obviously, the 1-day-exposure to light accelerated the progress of the disease.

One is tempted to assume that this detrimental effect of light is a manifestation of the hereditary abnormality. We were surprised, therefore, to find that heterozygous animals as well as *normal controls* were also severely affected by excessive light. In these experiments the rats were kept in cages surrounded by fluorescent circular lamps of 16-in diameter ("Circline G. E. 'Daylight White' or 4500° White"). Sheets of colored acrylic plastic (Plexiglass #2045, 2092, and 2444) were interposed between lamps and cage, and cooled by air. The animals were *albinos* of either sex (CDF or CDC (Charles River Farm)) or Sprague-Dawley on a "Wayne Lab-Blox" diet (Allied Mills, Inc., Chicago). Within the cage the animals behaved normally, periods of sleep (eyes closed) alternated with feeding and drinking. Retinal rhodopsin concentration measured immediately after one or more hours of exposure was used to estimate the intensity of retinal illumination; under conditions which affected the retina in the manner to be described retinal rhodopsin varied between 10 and 30% of the total present in the dark-adapted state.

The irreversible effects upon the ERG resulting from a 24-hr exposure to light are illustrated in Fig. 12. The ERGs of the control animals (*right column*), kept under the same conditions, but in the dark, are compared with those of animals exposed to green light, using Plexiglass #2092 (transmission range 490–580 mμ). Blue light equal in regard to bleaching or ERG stimulation produced approximately the same damage.

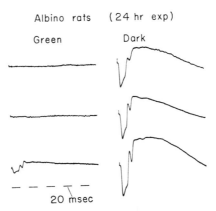

Albino rats   (24 hr exp)

Green   Dark

20 msec

FIG. 12. Effect of excessive light upon normal albino rats. Each ERG is from a different animal. Animals of right column were exposed to bright, green light for 24 hr; animals of left column were maintained under similar conditions as those of right column except for the interposition of a nontransmitting filter between lights and animals. The environmental temperature of both groups of animals was 38°C. The ERGs were tested 3–5 days after the exposure to light; the low amplitude ERGs were associated with massive histological damage.

The ERGs were recorded 3 days after exposure and were markedly reduced for most of the exposed animals; there was no recovery from any ERG reduction measured at this time. Subsequent histology (1–4 weeks after exposure) revealed that in the affected animals the visual cells had disappeared completely when the ERG had been extinct, or partially so when the ERG was only reduced. The inner retinal layers were unaffected but the retinal pigment epithelial cells were degenerated in the area of visual cell death. Similar effects were also observed with "normal", hooded animals (Long Evans strain).

The most important variable in determining the effectiveness of excessive light proved to be body (and eye) temperature; the higher body temperature, the greater the light induced damage. When the animals were kept at a rectal temperature of 104°F exposure to the light described above for 2–4 hr could completely destroy the visual cells. Increased body temperature in the dark or during red light was ineffective. We have not yet determined the action spectrum of this effect which obviously must be known before conclusions can be drawn. But whatever may turn out to be the molecule upon which light acts in this case, the effect clearly provides another example of the astounding vulnerability of the visual cells.

7. Concluding Remarks

It is tempting to assume that the specialized function of the visual cells, the transduction of light into excitation, basically determines their exceptional vulnerability and the manifestation of the genetic abnormality. Furthermore, one would like to assume that it is a specific cellular process governed by this specialized function on which visual cell viability depends to a much greater degree than that of other cells. On the basis of this reasoning, I cannot help but be impressed by the fact that excessive light destroys the visual cells and the pigment epithelium of albino as well as pigmented animals. Although nothing definite can be said at the present time, the effect reminds one of the so-called "photodynamic actions" of light (cf. Davson, 1960) which all seem to be photosensitized oxidations. Such oxidations one would expect to occur more readily in tissue which contains a light activated energy transfer system such as discussed in this symposium by Cohen and Noell. I therefore propose for consideration the thought that the specific vulnerability of the visual cells as evidenced by the effects of X-irradiation, O_2-poisoning and excessive light, is the manifestation of the ready occurrence of detrimental oxidizing reactions, perhaps because protective (antioxidant) mechanisms are very delicately poised.

REFERENCES

Babel, J. and Ziv, B. (1956). *Ophthalmologica Basel* **132**, 65.
Bourne, M. C., Campbell, D. A. and Tansley, K. (1938). *Br. J. Ophthal.* **22**, 613.
Brotherton, J. (1962). *Exp. Eye Res.* **1**, 234.
Brückner, R. (1951). *Docum. Ophthal.* **5–6**, 452.
Caravaggio, L. L. and Bonting, S. L. (1963). *Exp. Eye Res.* **2**, 12.
Cogan, D. G. (1950), *Trans. Am. Acad. Ophthal. Otolaryng.* 54th Meeting, V. p. 629.
Cohen, L. H. (1957). *Fed. Proc.* **16**, 165.
Cohen, L. and Noell, W. K. (1960). *J. Neurochem.* **5**, 253.
Davson, H. (1960). *Textbook of General Physiology*, Churchill, London.
DeRobertis, E. and Lasansky, A. (1961). In *The Structure of the Eye*, ed. by G. K. Smelser, pp. 29–49, Academic Press, New York.
DiPaolo, J. A. and Noell, W. K. (1962). Exp. Eye Res. **1**, 215.
Dowling, J. E. (1960). *Am. J. Ophthal.* **50**, 205.
Dowling, J. E. and Sidman, R. L. (1962). *J. Cell Biol.* **14**, 73.
Dowling, J. E. and Wald, G. (1960). *Proc. natn. Acad. Sci. U.S.A.* **46**, 587.
Gerschman, R., Gilbert, D. L., Nye, S. W., Dwyer, P. and Fenn, W. O. (1953). *Science* **119**, 623.
Graymore, C. (1960). *Br. J. Ophthal.* **44**, 363.
Graymore, C. (1964). *Nature Lond.*, **201**, 615.
Graymore, C., Tansley, K. and Kerly, M. (1959). *Biochem. J.* **72**, 459.
Gruneberg, H. (1943). *The Genetics of the Mouse*, Cambridge University Press, Cambridge.
Johnson, M. L. (1943). *Arch. Ophthal.* **29**, 793.
Karli, P. (1952). *Archs. Anat. Histol. Embryol.* **35**, 1.
Karli, P. (1963). *Adv. Ophthal.* **14**. 51.
Keeler, C. E. (1924). *Proc. natn. Acad. Sci. U.S.A.*, **10**, 329.
Lasansky, A. and DeRobertis, E. (1959). *J. biophys. biochem. Cytol.* **5**, 245.
Lowry, O. H., Roberts, N. R. and Lewis, G. (1956). *J. biol. Chem.* **220**, 879.
Lucas, D. R. J. (1958). *Embryol. Exp. Morph.* **65**, 589.
Noell, W. K. (1951). *J. cell. comp. Physiol.* **37**, 283.
Noell, W. K. (1953a). *Amer. J. Ophthal.* **36**, 103.
Noell, W. K. (1953b). *USAF SAM Project* #21–1201–004, pp. 1–22.
Noell, W. K. (1958). *Arch. Ophthal.* **60**, 702.
Noell, W. K. (1959). *Friedenwald Memorial Lecture*, *Am. J. Ophthal.* **48**, 347.
Noell, W. K. (1962a). In *Response of the Nervous System to Ionizing Radiation*, pp. 543–559. Academic Press, New York.
Noell, W. K. (1962b). In *Environmental Effects on Consciousness*, ed. by K. Schaeffer. McMillan Press, New York.
Noell, W. K. (1963). *J. opt. Soc. Am.* **53**, 36.
Noell, W. K., Crapper, D. R. and Paganelli, C. V. (1964). In *Transcellular Membrane Potentials and Ion Fluxes*, ed. by Snell and Noell, pp. 91–128. Gordon and Breach, New York.
Paigen, K. (1961a). *Proc. natn. Acad. Sci. U.S.A.* **47**, 1641.
Paigen, K. (1961b). *Exp. Cell Res.* **24**, 286.
Paigen, K. and Noell, W. K., (1961). *Nature, Lond.* **190**, 148.
Sorsby, A. (1941). *Br. J. Ophthal.* **25**, 58.

Sorsby, A. and Harding, R., (1960). *Nature, Lond.* **187**, 608.
Tansley, K. (1951). *Br. J. Ophthal.* **35**, 573–582.
Tansley, K. (1954). *J. Heredity* **45**, 123.
Trowell, O. A. (1954). *Exp. Cell Res.* **6**, 246.
Walters, P. T. (1960). *Br. J. Ophthal.* **43**, 686.

Protein Biosynthesis and the Hexosemonophosphate Shunt in the Developing Normal and Dystrophic Retina

H. W. Reading

Wernher Research Unit on Ophthalmological Genetics, Royal College of Surgeons, London, England

The rate of protein synthesis was determined both *in vivo* and *in vitro* in the retinas of normal rats and rats affected with hereditary retinal dystrophy by measurement of the incorporation of [^{14}C]glycine into total protein. The retinal dystrophy is a recessively inherited condition resembling human retinitis pigmentosa.

Experiments were carried out on litter-mates irrespective of sex, over the age range 6–24 days (*in vitro*) and 8 days (*in vivo*). *In vitro*, retinal tissue was incubated for 2-hr-periods in a phosphate medium containing glucose together with ^{14}C-labelled glycine. *In vivo*, each animal received a subcutaneous injection of radioactive glycine in isotonic saline.

In vitro, dystrophic retinas showed a significantly lower rate of glycine incorporation into protein than normal retinas at 6 and 8 days of age ($P=0.04$). At 10–16 days, differences, though present, were less marked ($P=0.07-0.30$) until at 24 days, incorporation rates were equal in both strains. Values for amino acid utilization and intracellular (amino acid pool) concentration of free [^{14}C]glycine after incubation were not significantly different in normal compared with affected tissues during the earlier stages, but at 24 days intracellular glycine concentration was markedly lower in the dystrophic retina.

In vivo, following injection of labelled glycine dystrophic retinas showed a marked depression in incorporation of amino acid compared with the normal. In addition, a depression in rate of protein degradation was observed. No differences were found in amino acid transport between normal and dystrophic animals.

In an earlier investigation glucose catabolism *via* the glycolytic and Krebs cycle pathways was studied in both normal and dystrophic retinas. Any quantitative changes detected were subsequent to histological degeneration of the affected retina. On the other hand, the anomaly in protein synthesis occurs some 6–8 days before histological changes can be detected. This depression of protein synthesis and turnover in the affected retina suggests an early discrepancy in production of an important cellular protein fraction, possibly with structural as well as functional properties. In the mammalian retina, an obvious candidate fulfilling these characteristics is the visual pigment, rhodopsin, or at least its protein moiety, opsin.

The hexose monophosphate (HMP) shunt pathway of glucose catabolism has been implicated in the normal functioning of the visual cycle in the mammalian retina. In consequence, it was decided to investigate the activity of this alternative pathway of glucose oxidation in developing normal and dystrophic retinas. This was carried out *in vitro* by measuring the incorporation of ^{14}C into respiratory CO_2 produced by incubating retinal tissue with specifically labelled glucose substrates. The results obtained showed striking differences between normal and dystrophic retinas in the degree of relative activity of the HMP shunt during retinal development. In the normal, non-functional retina, at 6–8 days of age, the HMP shunt activity is relatively high but activity decreases as development proceeds. On the other hand, HMP shunt activity in the dystrophic retina is about double that of the normal throughout early development and progression of the lesion.

The evidence available suggests an early anomaly in some control mechanism, which, in the normal retina, brings about a progressive decrease in HMP shunt activity. Knowledge of such mechanisms in mammalian tissue is lacking, although it is apparent that the activity of the HMP shunt is closely linked to the relative proportions of the reduced and oxidized forms of NADP (TPN) present intracellularly. An enzymatic mechanism coupled to the HMP shunt, having an obligatory requirement for NADP and involving oxido-reduction reactions, could be missing or reduced in content in the dystrophic tissue.

1. Introduction

Progressive hereditary degeneration of the retina, in conditions resembling human retinitis pigmentosa, has been the major subject of investigation at the Wernher Research Unit for the past 14 years. The studies have comprised histological and biochemical investigations and also the experimental induction of retinal degeneration.

Histology of retinal dystrophy

Histological studies by Sorsby, Koller, Attfield, Davey and Lucas (1954) on the Brückner strain of mice (Brückner, 1951) established that the retinal degeneration in these animals developed subsequently to differentiation into cellular layers, but before final differentiation of the rods had occurred—the earliest signs of this degeneration becoming apparent at about 10 days after birth. Similar findings were observed in the rat with retinal degeneration described by Bourne, Campbell and Tansley in 1938, and in the Irish setter described by Sorsby in 1941, the histological studies being recorded by Bourne et al. (1938) and Lucas, Attfield and Davey (1955) for the rat, and by Lucas (1954) for the Irish setter. In the rat and the dog, retinal degeneration sets in by about 12 days after birth, though, as in the mouse, full differentiation of the rods does not occur until about 21–28 days. The recessive hereditary character of the condition was established in all three species. In contrast to the view that hereditary degeneration in these animals supervenes in fully developed tissue—i.e., that these conditions are 'abiotrophies'—Sorsby and his associates have stressed that the lesion occurred in retina that had not developed fully. The retina, in fact, had never developed normally. They suggested the term dystrophy rather than abiotrophy for these disorders for in the affected animals the retina was already degenerate well before the neuro-epithelium had reached full differentiation in the normal. These observations opened up the possibility of studying the nature of the failure of the rods to become fully differentiated.

Electronmicroscopy

Electronmicroscopy of the dystrophic mouse retina by Lasansky and De Robertis (1960) confirmed these findings as regards the failure of the rod to develop fully and showed that the outer segment of the rod in the normal animals proceeds from a primitive cilium to the formation of membranous material which is re-orientated into sacs, finally building up into a definite regularly-layered structure. In the dystrophic mouse, anomalous changes occur in the re-orientation stage and the regularly layered structure never appears; instead degeneration takes place.

Similar studies by Dowling and Sidman (1962) on the rat showed the first sign of disease at 12 days of age as the accumulation of extra outer-segment like lamellae between the ends of the developing rods and the pigment epithelium. By 22 days, the inner segments and some photoreceptor cell nuclei are degenerate and the ERG shows diminished sensitivity.

Electroretinography

It is uncertain whether the retinal lesion in the mouse differs in a fundamental manner from that in the rat and the dog. In the mouse, the ERG is always abnormal (Noell, 1958) whereas in the rat the ERG develops to a virtually normal adult state and then becomes abnormal (Dowling and Sidman, 1962). In the dog, an ERG of an apparently adult type has been recorded (Parry, Tansley and Thomson, 1955).

Experimental degeneration of the retina

Following the observation by Sorsby (1941) that a single, intravenous injection of sodium iodate produces an acute degeneration of the neuro-epithelium and pigment layer of the retina, an extensive series of investigations have been carried out by Sorsby and his associates (Sorsby, Newhouse and Lucas, 1957; Sorsby and Nakajima, 1958; Sorsby and Harding, 1960, 1962) to determine the nature of the retinotoxic action of sodium iodate, iodoacetate, bromoacetate, a group of diamino diphenoxyalkanes, sodium fluoride and the diabetogenic agent, dithizone, and the bearing of these lesions on the hereditary dystrophy. They also explored the possibility of protecting the retina from experimentally induced damage, and showed that certain aliphatic thiol compounds, in particular cysteine, did protect the retina against the toxic effect of iodate, but not against the action of any of the other retinotoxic compounds (Sorsby and Harding, 1962). The protective effect of cysteine appears to reside in chemical antagonism to iodate (Sorsby and Reading, 1964). The action of iodate and possibly some at least of the other retino-toxic agents appears to depend on the ability to disrupt the protein molecule with liberation of –SH groups.

2. Biochemical Investigation

The dependence of the retina on carbohydrate for its energy supply suggested that investigation of the metabolism of this food material might prove profitable, especially during the period of critical development of rod cell growth. Graymore, Tansley and Kerly (1959) found anaerobic glycolysis in the affected retina virtually unaltered from the normal until the 3rd week of life. They could not establish any relationship between anaerobic glycolytic activity and visual cell degeneration. Walters (1959) and Brotherton (1960) also reported a decline in the rate of anaerobic glycolysis in affected retinas, but again this effect was not markedly apparent until 16–25 days of age.

Investigation of aerobic glucose metabolism *via* Embden-Meyerhof and Krebs cycle pathways by Reading and Sorsby (1962) revealed no qualitative differences between normal and dystrophic retinas, such quantitative differences which were detectable being subsequent to histological degeneration. However, it was found that the dystrophic retina, unlike its normal counterpart, failed to retain intracellularly, some of the amino acids formed directly from the carbon skeleton of glucose. This 'leakage' of amino acids suggested a possible effect on protein biosynthesis, so that investigation of the uptake, transport and incorporation into retinal protein of labelled amino acid both *in vivo* and *in vitro*, was undertaken. An early depression in rate of protein synthesis in the dystrophic retina was discovered (Reading and Sorsby, 1964). Recent work had indicated the existence of a parallelism between rate of protein synthesis and activity of the hexose monophosphate shunt pathway (HMP) of glucose catabolism (Beaconsfield and Reading, 1964) so it was decided to evaluate the relative importance of the HMP shunt in normal and dystrophic retinas.

3. Materials and Methods

Animals and preparation of tissues

Pink-eyed piebald agouti rats, affected with the retinal dystrophy (Bourne et al., 1938) and for comparison, black-hooded (PVG) rats were used throughout the series. All experiments were carried out on litter-mates irrespective of sex. Retinas were prepared for biochemical experiments by keeping them immersed in ice-cold physiological saline while carrying out dissection. Where necessary, wet weights of retinal tissue were determined on a torsion balance after removing surplus liquid.

Incubation conditions for protein biosynthesis

Uniformly labelled [^{14}C]glycine (obtained from the Radiochemical Centre, Amersham, England) with a specific activity of 2·19 mc/mM was added to the incubation medium in amounts which brought the activity in each flask to 5·0 μc. Incubations in 1 ml Krebs-Ringer phosphate medium (Dawson, Elliot, Elliot and Jones, 1959) using about 25 mg (wet wt) quantities of retinal tissue were carried out using 5 ml micro-Warburg flask in a conventional Warburg apparatus. The gas phase was pure oxygen. Non-radioactive glucose was added to give a final concentration in the medium of 0·1%.

As quickly as possible after dissection, the retinal tissue was added to previously chilled Warburg flasks, which were then gassed and equilibrated at 37°C. Commencement of reaction was taken as the time of tipping radioactive glycine from the side-arm into the main compartment.

Incubation was continued for 2 hr at 37° whereupon the flasks and contents were rapidly chilled and the retinal protein fractionated by a method similar to that of Siekevitz (1952).

Incubation conditions for HMP shunt determinations

Twenty-five mg quantities of retinal tissue were incubated at 37° in 1 ml Krebs-Ringer bicarbonate medium (Dawson et al., 1959) in an atmosphere of 95% oxygen, 5% carbon dioxide, in special micro-Warburg flasks, fitted with two side-arms, one of which was closed with a rubber vaccine cap. Two μc of either [1–^{14}C]glucose or [6–^{14}C]glucose, diluted with inert carrier glucose to give a final concentration of 0·1% in the medium, was added from the side-arm to initiate the reaction. Reaction was stopped at the end of 1 hr-incubation by injecting acid into the medium. This also served to drive off dissolved carbon dioxide which was collected on paper rolls in the centre-well, the paper having been soaked with alkali (by injection) just prior to introducing acid.

Fractionation procedure and measurement of radioactivity

Fractionation of the retinal protein consisted of homogenizing the retina following incubation and extracting with 10% trichloracetic acid (TCA), followed by removal of nucleic acids and lipids from the precipitated protein. Radioactivity of the dried protein residues was measured by dissolving the protein pellets in 98% formic acid and plating the solution on aluminium planchets using lens tissue to obtain an even film. Planchets were dried in vacuum over KOH and the amount of protein determined by weighing on a micro-balance. The possibility that radioactivity in the protein samples could arise from adsorbed radioactive amino acid was eliminated by subjecting aliquots of the protein precipitates to ninhydrin-carbon dioxide degradation (van Slyke, MacFadyen and Hamilton, 1941).

Radioactive carbon dioxide collected on the KOH papers in the HMP shunt experiments was precipitated as barium carbonate, plated out and dried. All radioactivity determinations of 'solid' material on planchets were made under a thin end-window Geiger-Müller counter, suitable corrections being made for self-absorption, etc.

Individual figures of results for [^{14}C]glycine uptake and incorporation are averages from 6 to 9 litters with 8-10 rats per litter.

Treatment of medium and extracts

Aliquots of incubation medium and TCA extracts were chromatographed on Whatman no. 1 paper, using the bi-dimensional system (a) Sec-butanol 75·0 ml, formic acid (85%) 14·5 ml, water 15·5 ml, (b) phenol (redistilled) 80 g, water 20 ml, ammonia (0·880) 1·0 ml.

In the HMP shunt experiments, glucose substrate remaining in the incubation medium was characterized by paper chromatography on Whatman no. 1 paper in a solvent system of tert-butanol 80 ml, picric acid 4·0 g, water 20 ml. Radioactivity of the developed spots on all chromatograms was evaluated in an automatic scanning device (Frank, Chain, Pocchiari and Rossi, 1959).

Conditions for in vivo *determinations of retinal protein synthesis*

In this series of experiments, 8-day-old littermates of either normal or dystrophic rats were injected subcutaneously with a saline solution of uniformly ^{14}C-labelled glycine, at a dose of 10 μc per animal. Animals were killed in pairs at intervals after injection, the retinas removed, homogenized and extracted in cold 10% TCA. Subsequent steps, ending in the counting of retinal protein, were exactly as described for the *in vitro* experiments. Livers were also removed from each animal, washed in saline, blotted dry, weighed and homogenized in 2 × 5 ml quantities of cold 10% TCA, then treated as for retina.

4. Results

Protein biosynthesis in the retina

Uptake and content of [^{14}C]glycine in the amino acid pool

Figure 1 shows the uptake of [^{14}C]glycine from the incubation medium. Rates of uptake in both normal and affected retinas are virtually equal. At equilibrium, the level of radioactivity in tissue extracts (Fig. 2) is a measure of the amount of glycine

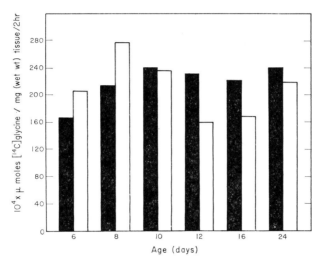

Fig. 1. Uptake of [^{14}C]glycine from incubation medium. The significance of the differences between the mean values was in no case higher than $P = 0.2$. In this and following figures black columns represent normal animals, and white columns those of the dystrophic rat.

in the intracellular amino acid pool. This is a measure of the rate of transport of glycine and it can be seen in all cases except one, that there was no significant difference between normal and dystrophic retinas. In the later stages of the lesion, the intracellular glycine concentration was lowered in the dystrophic tissue.

Rate of protein biosynthesis

Figure 3 illustrates the incorporation of [^{14}C]glycine into retinal protein based on the relative specific activities of the dried protein samples. At 6 and 8 days of age, incorporation rates were significantly lower ($P = 0.04$) in dystrophic retina than in the normal. Although a difference was maintained at later ages, viz., 10–24 days, the significance of the differences from normal became progressively lower, until at 24 days, incorporation rates were virtually the same in both normal and affected retinas.

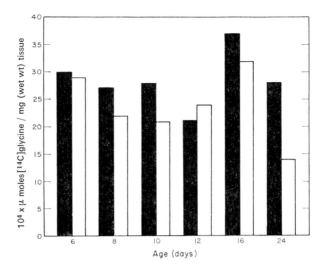

F<small>IG</small>. 2. Concentration of free [^{14}C]glycine in trichloracetic acid extracts of retinas following incubation. The significance of the differences between the mean values varied from $P = 0\cdot6$ to $P = 0\cdot8$ over the period 6–16 days. At 24 days significance was higher $P = 0\cdot02$.

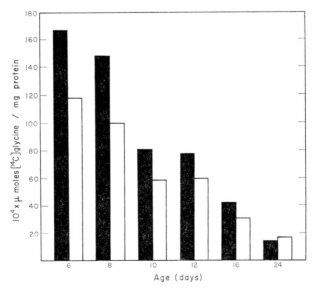

F<small>IG</small>. 3. Incorporation of [^{14}C]glycine into retinal protein in vitro. Significance of the differences between the mean values was as follows: 6 days $P = 0\cdot04$, 8 days $0\cdot04 > P > 0\cdot02$, 10 days $0\cdot07 > P > 0\cdot05$, 12 days $P = 0\cdot1$, 16 days $P = 0\cdot3$, 24 days $P = 0\cdot4$.

The amino acid incorporation figures, taken as a series, show the pattern of a definite difference in rates of protein biosynthesis at an early age, with this difference diminishing in size as development proceeds.

In vivo *experiments with 8-day-old rats*

Figure 4 shows the concentration of [^{14}C]glycine in TCA extracts of retinal tissue following injection of the labelled amino acid. No real difference in amino acid transport into the retina between normal and dystrophic animals was found, so confirming the *in vitro* results.

Figure 5 presents the results of determinations of *in vivo* incorporation of [^{14}C] glycine into retinal protein in normal and dystrophic rats. A small and probably

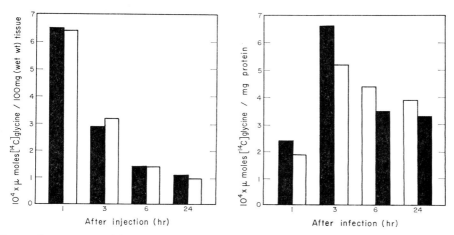

Fig. 4. Concentration of free [^{14}C]glycine in trichloracetic acid extracts of retina following injection of labelled amino acid (10 μc per animal). Each value represents the mean of 3 or 4 determinations.

Fig. 5. *In vivo* incorporation of [^{14}C]glycine into retinal protein following injection of labelled amino acid (10 μc per animal). Each value represents the mean of 4 determinations.

insignificant difference was recorded 1 hr after injection, but after 3 hr, the higher rate of incorporation in the normal animal was quite marked. In contrast, however, 6 and 24 hr after injection, dystrophic animals showed higher values for incorporation of labelled amino acid, which would indicate a slower rate of turnover than in the corresponding normal retina.

Figure 6 shows comparative results for glycine incorporation into liver protein

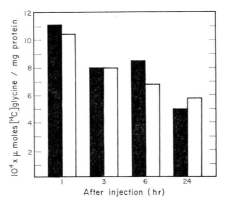

Fig. 6. *In vivo* incorporation of [^{14}C]glycine into liver protein following injection of labelled amino acid (10 μc per animal). Each value represents the mean of 4 determinations.

of normal and dystrophic animals. No marked differences were apparent between the two strains.

Hexose monophosphate shunt activity in normal and dystrophic retinas

Evaluation of the relative activity of the HMP shunt for glucose breakdown was carried out by expressing the yields of $^{14}CO_2$ (called specific yields) in terms of the corresponding glucose substrate utilized. This method of presenting the results is based on the suggestions of Katz and Wood (1963) and overcomes the difficulties encountered when yields of $^{14}CO_2$ alone, without any reference to the amount of substrate which may be utilized in parallel experiments, are compared for the evaluation of HMP shunt activity.

In all cases, the activities of the carbon dioxide collected, were calculated to conform to a constant specific activity of glucose substrate, the latter being determined on samples of medium before incubation.

In dystrophic retinas, over the age range 6–28 days, the activity of the HMP shunt pathway is appreciably higher than in corresponding normal retinas (Table I).

TABLE I

Activity of the hexose monophosphate shunt in normal and dystrophic rat retinas

Age	Normal	Dystrophic	% increase in dystrophic	
6–7 days	2·9 (0·6)	4·1 (0·8)	41%	$0.37 > P > 0.2$
14 days	1·7 (0·3)	2·5 (0·6)	49%	$0.2 > P > 0.1$
27–28 days	1·2 (0·1)	1·8 (0·2)	50%	$0.05 > P > 0.02$

(S.E.M. in parenthesis)

Results expressed as: $\dfrac{\text{Specific yield } ^{14}CO_2 \text{ from } [1\text{–}^{14}C] \text{ glucose}}{\text{Specific yield } ^{14}CO_2 \text{ from } [6\text{–}^{14}C] \text{ glucose}}$.

The differences, however, are greater and show higher statistical significance during the later stages of development of the lesion. The results obtained also demonstrate the decline in relative importance of the shunt pathway for glucose catabolism which occurs with increase in age and development in the normal retina.

5. Discussion

Difference in incorporation of [^{14}C] glycine in normal and dystrophic retinas

The amino acid incorporation experiments have shown that the immature, developing retina has a high initial rate of protein synthesis, this rate decreasing with increase in age until a steady turnover is established after the tissue has become more or less fully differentiated. The situation in the retina is very similar to that observed by Richter (1955) in mammalian brain during foetal development.

The lowered rate of protein synthesis in the dystrophic retina, both *in vitro* and *in vivo*, is markedly apparent before differentiation of the tissue has begun. At later stages, differences between normal and affected retinas are not so apparent. The anomaly in protein synthesis in the dystrophic retina occurs at least 6–8 days before any damage to the visual cells can be detected histologically. This is an extremely important observation since it follows the pattern of other genetically controlled abnormalities in which protein synthesis or protein structure have been implicated (Harris,

1963; Marks and Burka, 1964). *In vivo*, there was evidence of a slower rate of protein degradation as well as of synthesis in the dystrophic retina. This is not incompatible with established ideas on protein metabolism since it is known that conditions which reduce protein synthesis, also reduce its breakdown (Campbell, 1958).

Alteration in amino acid transport does not appear to be a contributory factor for the depressed rate of protein synthesis, since both *in vitro* and *in vivo* experiments show that the influx of glycine into either normal or dystrophic retinas was virtually equal. It would appear, therefore, that the anomaly in protein synthesis is not due to a breakdown in energy-utilization processes, which was earlier thought to be a possibility.

The nature of the protein anomaly in the dystrophic retina

The anomaly in protein synthesis in the immature, dystrophic retina is most likely a manifestation of an inadequate or "abnormal" synthesis of a specific protein entity, either enzymatic or structural in character. Inadequate general protein synthesis is unlikely, since the dystrophic retina grows and develops normally except that at the end of the differentiation period, rod cell outer segments do not develop fully and begin to degenerate followed by general degeneration of the visual cell layer.

Role of the HMP shunt in normal and dystrophic retinas

The significance of the elevation in HMP shunt activity is not immediately apparent although it is noteworthy that the effect follows the protein anomaly in the time-course of the lesion. In fact, the depression in rate of protein synthesis in the dystrophic retina decreases in relative intensity while at the same time, the elevation in HMP shunt activity is increasing. The shunt pathway for glucose oxidation has been implicated in the normal functioning of the visual cycle in the mammalian retina by some recent elegant researches of Futterman (1963). After bleaching, reduction of retinene to vitamin A alcohol by retinene reductase is coupled to the shunt by utilization of $NADPH_2$, produced by shunt oxidations. It would appear that some mechanism which has an influence or control on shunt activity is affected in the dystrophic retina as a consequence of the anomaly in protein synthesis.

Significance of the experimental findings

Amongst the various oxido-reduction enzyme systems which are metabolically coupled with the shunt, the $NADP/NADPH_2$ retinene reductase (alcohol dehydrogenase) system has the closest association with retinal function. Evidence has recently been presented for *in vitro* systems (Beaconsfield and Reading, 1964) that endogenous HMP shunt activity in numerous tissues can be controlled by alterations in concentration of the $NADP/NADPH_2$-alcohol dehydrogenase system and that the activities of the two enzyme systems are in inverse proportion to each other. Since the HMP shunt is stimulated in the dystrophy, retinene reductase (alcohol dehydrogenase) activity is likely to be reduced. This suggestion is under experimental verification.

What is not clear however, is the point at which actual structural breakdown occurs as a result of the biochemical lesion and why such structural breakdown should result from say, an enzyme deficiency. Regarding retinene reductase, Futterman and Saslaw (1961) first drew attention to the close intracellular localization of this enzyme and rhodopsin; both reside in the highly insoluble particulate fraction following very high speed centrifugation of rod segments. There may be some physico-chemical interdependence between these two proteins such that any change in one, affects the other.

F

REFERENCES

Beaconsfield, P. and Reading, H. W. (1964). *Nature, Lond.* **202**, 464.

Bourne, M. C., Campbell, D. A. and Tansley, K. (1938). *Br. J. Ophthal.* **22**, 613.

Brotherton, J. (1960), Birmingham University. Ph.D. Thesis.

Brückner, R. (1951). Docum. Ophthal. **5–6**, 452.

Campbell, P. N. (1958). *Advances in Cancer Research*, Volume 5, p. 98. Academic Press, New York.

Dawson, R. M. C., Elliott, D. C., Elliott, W. H. and Jones, K. M. (1959). *Data for Biochemical Research*. Clarendon Press, Oxford.

Dowling, J. E. and Sidman, R. L. (1962). *J. Cell Biol.* **14**, 73.

Frank, M., Chain, E. B., Pocchiari, F. and Rossi, C. (1959). *Selected Scientific Papers*. Istituto Superiore di Sanita, **2**, 75.

Futterman, S. (1963). *J. biol. Chem.* **238**, 1145.

Futterman, S. and Saslaw, L. D. (1961). *J. biol. Chem.* **236**, 1652.

Graymore, C. N., Tansley, K. and Kerley, M. (1959). *Biochem. J.* **72**, 459.

Harris, H. (1963). *Garrod's Inborn Errors of Metabolism*. Oxford University Press, London.

Katz, J. and Wood, H. G. (1963). *J. biol. Chem.* **238**, 517.

Lasansky, A. and De Robertis, E. (1960). *J. biophys. biochem. Cytol.* **7**, 679.

Lucas, D. R. (1954). *J. exp. Zool.* **126**, 537.

Lucas, D. R., Attfield, M. and Davey, J. B. (1955). *J. Path. Bact.* **70**, 469.

Marks, P. A. and Burka, E. R. (1964). *Science* **144**, 552.

Noell, W. K. (1958). *Arch. Ophthal.* **60**, 725.

Parry, H. B., Tansley, K. and Thomson, L. C. (1955). *Br. J. Ophthal.* **39**, 349.

Reading, H. W. and Sorsby, A. (1962). *Vision Res.* **2**, 315.

Reading, H. W. and Sorsby, A. (1964). *Biochem. J.* **90**, 38P.

Richter, D. (1955). In *Biochemistry of the Developing Nervous System*, ed. by H. Waelsch, p. 241. Academic Press, New York.

Siekevitz, P. (1952). *J. biol. Chem.* **195**, 549.

van Slyke, D. D., MacFadyen, D. A. and Hamilton, P. (1941). *J. biol. Chem.*, **141**, 671.

Sorsby, A. (1941). *Br. J. Ophthal.* **25**, 58.

Sorsby, A. and Harding, R. (1960). *Br. J. Ophthal.* **44**, 213.

Sorsby, A. and Harding, R. (1962). *Vision Res.* **2**, 149.

Sorsby, A. and Harding, R. (1962). *Vision Res.* **2**, 139.

Sorsby, A., Koller, P. C., Attfield, M., Davey, J. B. and Lucas, D. R. (1954). *J. exp. Zool.* **125**, 171.

Sorsby, A. and Nakajima, A. (1958). *Br. J. Ophthal.* **42**, 563.

Sorsby, A., Newhouse, J. P. and Lucas, D. R. (1957). *Br. J. Ophthal.* **41**, 39.

Sorsby, A. and Reading, H. W. (1964). *Vision Res.* (1964) **4**, 51.

Walters, P. T. (1959). *Br. J. Ophthal.* **43**, 686.

Further Comments on the Metabolism of the Retina of the Normal and 'Retinitis' Rat during Development

CLIVE N. GRAYMORE

Department of Pathology, Institute of Ophthalmology, University of London, England

This communication reports recent studies in the author's laboratory dealing with glucose metabolism in the retina of the normal and 'retinitis' rat during development. Particular attention is paid to the activity of the pentose phosphate pathway and the isoenzyme patterns of lactic acid dehydrogenase.

Although a great deal is known as regards the gross metabolism of the retina, the assignation of specific biochemical properties to the individual components of the retina continues to provide a challenge to the investigator. A variety of techniques have been employed to assist our understanding of the metabolic differentiation of this tissue, including conventional histochemistry (Cogan and Kuwabara, 1959; Kuwabara and Cogan, 1959, 1960; Berkow and Patz, 1961a,b; see also Kuwabara, this Symposium) ultramicrodissection coupled with quantitative histochemical procedures (Lowry, Roberts and Lewis, 1956) and the study of metabolic patterns in both the retina of the normal animal during development as well as those occurring as a result of either chemically-induced or naturally-occurring degenerations. This last situation has been reviewed most adequately (Cohen and Noell, Noell and Potts, this Symposium).

In view of the nature of the two previous papers, however, it seems opportune at this stage to refer briefly to some of the more recent findings of my own laboratory.

At one stage whilst studying the metabolic development of the normal rat retina, Dr. Mary Towlson and I became interested in the role played by the pentose phosphate route. The techniques employed were conventional and involved measuring the extent of oxidation *in vitro* of the C-1 and C-6 of appropriately labelled [^{14}C]glucose (Graymore and Towlson, 1965a). The results obtained showed that the ratio of oxidation of C-1/C-6 by the mature rat retina is 1·13, a result that compares favourably with the values obtained by other workers (see Table I). The assumption that, under

TABLE I

C-1/C-6 Ratio of normal adult retina

Futterman and Kinoshita, 1959a (ox)	..	..	..	1·20
Cohen and Noell, 1960 (rabbit)	..	..	..	1·14
Rahman and Kerly, 1961 (ox) ..	..	..	..	1·30
Graymore and Towlson, 1964 (rat)	..	..	..	1·13

the conditions defined, this relatively low ratio implies minimal 'shunt' activity in the mature retina is generally accepted (but see Katz and Wood, 1960, 1963, for theoretical limitations). In the case of the retina excised from the 7-day-old ratling this ratio is increased (Table II). The results are expressed as total cts/min per retina, it having been established that within experimental limits the specific activity of the C-1 and C-6 labelled media were the same. Previous work from a number of laboratories has shown that the metabolic activity of the 'immature' retina, when judged in terms of glucose metabolism, is considerably lower than that of the adult, representing in the rat, for example, approximately one-third of that of the mature animal

TABLE II

Radioactive counts obtained from C-1- and C-6-labelled glucose

	C-1-labelled glucose		C-6-labelled glucose		C-1-labelled glucose + phenazine methosulphate		C-1/C-6	Increase in the capacity of the hexose mono-phosphate shunt with phenazine	No. of assays
	cts/min /retina	cts/min /mg prot.	cts/min /retina	cts/min /mg prot.	cts/min /retina	cts/min /mg prot.			
Normal adult rat	2867	1874	2540	1660	4988	3260	1·13	74%	6
7-day ratling	556	561	372	375	3976	4015	1·49	715%	4

Average dry weight of normal adult retina is taken as 1·53 mg protein.
Average dry weight of 7-day ratling retina is taken as 0·99 mg protein.

when expressed on the basis of activity per mg protein (Graymore, 1960). The figures in Table I reveal that during development there is a 3·3-fold increase in C-1 oxidation, contrasting with a 4·4-fold increase in C-6 oxidation, these unequal changes being reflected as an increased ratio of C-1/C-6 of 1·49 in the 'immature' retina. It would seem, therefore, that although the activity of the pentose phosphate pathway is low in both the 'immature' and the 'mature' retina, the activity of this pathway is higher, relatively, in the retina of the young rat. This finding, again, is in accordance with the observations of Cohen and Noell (1960) for the rabbit. It is tempting to assume that the higher relative activity of the shunt mechanism in the retina of the immature animal is associated with biosynthetic pathways essential to the tissue differentiation required for normal development.

There are, however, other ways of investigating the activity of the 'shunt' pathway. One can, for example, measure the levels of the oxidised and reduced forms of the pyridine nucleotides. The evidence obtained in this way is probably more circumstantial than that obtained from C-1/C-6 studies but carries the merit of determining absolute values as they exist *in vivo*; the retina is removed within 1-2 min of anaesthesis and frozen in liquid nitrogen. The complications of interpreting the results of either procedure have been stressed many times, however, but the combination of both approaches would appear to be most advantageous in investigations of this kind.

The levels of these coenzymes in the retina were first measured by Slater, Heath and Graymore (1962) and found to bear a striking resemblance to those found in brain (Lowry, Passonneau, Schulz and Rock, 1961), but to differ markedly from those of liver (Slater and Sawyer, 1962). The relatively low ratio of $NADPH_2/NADP$ contrasted with the high ratio found in other tissues known to have an active pentose phosphate pathway (cf. Dumont, 1960) and seemed to endorse the view that although this 'shunt' mechanism can occur in the adult retina, it does not appear to play a prominent role. Dr. Towlson and I repeated these estimations more recently, and extended the investigations to the levels in the retina of the immature rat (Graymore and Towlson, 1965a). The results we obtained showed that the total oxidized and reduced pyridine nucleotides increased by about 20% during the period of investigation (Table III), although the ratio $NAD + NADH_2/NADP + NADPH_2$ does not

TABLE III

Pyridine nucleotide levels of normal adult and immature rat retinas

Rats	NAD	$NADH_2$	Total $NAD+NADH_2$	$NAD/NADH_2$	$NADH_2/$ $NADPH_2$	No. of assays
Adult	$191\cdot8\pm4\cdot5$	$26\cdot6\pm1\cdot3$	$218\cdot4\pm4\cdot5$	$7\cdot21$	$1\cdot42$	11
Immature (6-7 day ratling)	$163\cdot9\pm7\cdot9$	$15\cdot1\pm1\cdot9$	$179\cdot0\pm5\cdot0$	$10\cdot85$	$0\cdot90$	8

	NADP	$NADPH_2$	Total $NADP+NADPH_2$	$NADPH_2/NADP$		
Adult	$4\cdot8\pm0\cdot6$	$18\cdot7\pm0\cdot6$	$23\cdot5\pm0\cdot4$	$3\cdot90$		11
Immature (6-7 day ratling)	$3\cdot1\pm0\cdot6$	$16\cdot8\pm0\cdot8$	$19\cdot9\pm0\cdot7$	$5\cdot40$		8

All nucleotide values are expressed in terms of $\mu g/g$ wet wt of retinal tissue. The calculations were based on a wet wt of $12\cdot8$ mg for the adult tissue and $8\cdot28$ mg for the immature.

change appreciably. The only significant change is in the redox state of the nucleotides; NAD is maintained in a more oxidized state in the 'immature' retina, whereas the NADP system is more reduced. This is reflected in a developmental decrease in the $NAD/NADH_2$ ratio from $10\cdot8$ to $7\cdot2$ and the $NADPH_2/NADP$ ratio from $5\cdot4$ to $3\cdot9$.

The difficulties inherent in attempting to attribute significance to these findings have been emphasized many times, and certain generalizations discussed (see Graymore and Towlson, 1965a). It seems, however, that the retina falls into line with other tissues in the respect that the reduced form of the NADP system, and the oxidized form of the NAD system invariably predominate. This is in accord with the general assumption that in biosynthetic pathways a reaction involving reduction is associated with $NADPH_2$, whereas during oxidation the pyridine nucleotide most frequently involved is NAD.

The assumption that a high ratio of $NADPH_2/NADP$ imputes high activity to the pentose phosphate pathway is, however, open to doubt. The correlation is based on empirical evidence, and the concept would not apply if the availability of NADP were the rate limiting step. This poses something of a problem in the retina, for evidence from radioactive studies (*vide supra*) argues in favour of this relatively higher ratio of $NADPH_2/NADP$ being compatible with raised activity of the pentose phosphate pathway. On the other hand, the addition of artificial electron acceptors, such as phenazine methosulphate, to the *in vitro* system stimulates the oxidation of C-1 to a considerable degree (Table II; Cohen and Noell, 1960; Graymore and Towlson, 1965).

This endorses the view that the availability of suitable electron acceptors might be a rate-limiting-factor in the retina as regards control of the 'shunt' mechanism. There is little doubt, however, that the interpretation of the significance of the levels of the pyridine nucleotides is frequently oversimplified. They participate in a variety of metabolic sequences within the cell, and it is difficult to relate changes in their ratios with specific pathways. Futterman (1963), for example, has provided convincing evidence that $NADPH_2$ is the coenzyme of choice for retinal alcohol dehydrogenase, and it might well be argued that the morphological development of the visual cells, coupled with their associated capacity for light induced excitation would lead to a shift of emphasis in the NADP system towards the oxidized form during maturation. This would result in a fall of the $NADPH_2/NADP$ ratio during development as has been found. Until more is learned of the comparative quantitative roles of the different systems it is difficult to assess the significance of the observed changes.

At the time that Dr. Towlson and myself were involved in these studies I became interested, largely from the clinical standpoint, in the electrophoretic separation of lactic acid dehydrogenase into its constituent isoenzymes (Graymore, 1964a,b). Futterman and Kinoshita (1959b), applying zone electrophoresis on starch paste, had isolated 5 fractions of this enzyme from the retina. I applied the more rapid and simpler procedure of cellulose acetate electrophoresis to the same analysis and confirmed their results, inasmuch as there were 5 fractions which reacted with either NAD or NADP, although the activity of all the fractions was higher with the former coenzyme.

These studies were extended to an analysis of the isoenzyme pattern of the developing retina of both the normal and 'retinitis pigmentosa' rat, and the results are summarized in Fig. 1.* During the course of these studies, an essentially similar but

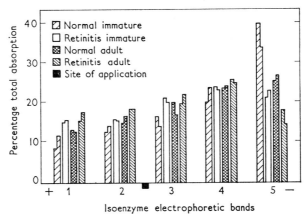

Fig. 1. Absorption of 5 isoenzymes of LDH expressed as a percentage of total and extracted from retinas of normal and retinitis rats during development.

quite independent investigation was being carried out by Bonavita, Ponte and Amore (1963) using the technique of starch gel electrophoresis. Professor Bonavita has described his findings in detail in this Symposium, so I will confine myself to a brief summary of my conclusions. Figure 1 shows that LDH 5, corresponding to the so-called 'muscle' (M) isoenzyme of other workers, is substantially reduced in both the immature and mature 'retinitis' retina when compared to that of a normal animal. The existence of this early deviation from normality appears most exciting

*See Graymore, 1964b, for details.

as it suggests the possibility of a genetically controlled abberation evidencing itself some time before 'visible' degeneration. I stress *'visible'* degeneration, because it seems rather futile to refer to *biochemical* abnormalities occurring before *structural* damage. This is a matter of definition of terms, and relates to the molecular size in which we are dealing. The first metabolic error that occurs must represent the primary 'structural' change, and I agree with Professor Bonavita's statement yesterday that one can only continue to search for the earliest discernible change. We may then be able to differentiate between cause and effect.

The immediate problem from my point of view was to find some hypothesis on which to work, even should it prove to be false! The results had shown that in the normal animal, the anaerobic 'muscle' isoenzyme was most active in the immature retina, at a time when tissue differentiation was most marked. My results differed in this respect from those of Professor Bonavita and his colleagues. This was of interest inasmuch as the activity of the pentose phosphate pathway was also at peak level during this period, and both parameters fell during maturation. It is tempting, therefore, to speculate that this M isoenzyme, LDH 5, is responsible in some manner for driving this pathway which in turn plays some central role in the tissue differentiation. The most obvious means of accomplishing such a linkage would be by preferential usage of the appropriate coenzyme, but our results had confirmed those of Futterman and Kinoshita (1959) in demonstrating that no fraction differed from any other in its selectivity of coenzyme.

Evidence shows, however, that metabolic control is rather more subtle than can be shown on a conventional metabolic map! It has been established that many 'respiratory' enzymes may not be exclusively mitochondrial, and that the coenzyme requirement of individual enzymes is not as rigorously specific as at first thought. Electrophoretic studies in this laboratory have shown quite clearly, for example, that isocitrate dehydrogenase can occur in both the mitochondrial and soluble fractions of the rat retina. Differential centrifugation, and the examination of a high speed supernate by means of a modified technique based on the colorimetric determination of formazan production, have shown that an active NADP-dependent soluble isocitrate dehydrogenase exists in the retina (Graymore, unpublished results). It seems likely, when considering evidence from other tissues (see Dixon and Webb, 1958), that this system might well be coupled with the carbon dioxide fixing malic enzyme, also contained in the cell sap, and also being NADP-dependent. Rahman and Kerly (1961) investigated the effect of a bicarbonate buffer, as opposed to a phosphate buffer, on the oxidation of the C-1 and C-6 of glucose, on the assumption that the shunt mechanism might be involved in driving carbon dioxide fixation *via* the mutual coenzyme. Their failure to demonstrate a significant change might well be explained in the above terms.

It has been shown also in this laboratory that malic dehydrogenase exists both as a soluble and a mitochondrial fraction in the retina, and it would be most interesting to determine the respective roles played by these fractions in the sequence to the above mechanism. It seems, therefore, that there are a number of 'points systems' in these metabolic pathways that may well control and regulate the overall metabolic pattern. In this respect it is of importance that LDH 5(M) favours the conversion of pyruvate to lactate, whereas LDH 1, inhibited by increasing concentrations of pyruvate, assists entry of pyruvate into the Krebs cycle. Once again, a self adjusting

Note added in proof: Preliminary investigations have shown also that the LDH isoenzyme pattern of 'pure' outer limb preparations does not appear to differ from that of the whole tissue

points system operates, in this case to control the fate of pyruvate from the Embden Meyerhoff pathway. In the present context, it seems reasonable to suppose that regardless of any preferential usage of the NADP system by a particular isoenzyme fraction, the higher content of LDH 5 in the immature retina would favour the operation of the shunt by diverting a relatively greater proportion of pyruvate into lactic acid. A deficiency in this fraction in the 'retinitis' animal might interfere with the normal operation of this pathway and lead to a failure in normal differentiation.

Before concluding my comments, I would like to refer very briefly to the results of some investigations carried out over the last few weeks. It was thought that if the above hypothesis were true, the ratio of the oxidized and reduced forms of NADP should vary from normality in the retina of the 'retinitis' rats during the phase of degeneration. Table IV shows the results of these preliminary measurements, and it

TABLE IV

Levels of pyridine nucleotides in retinas of 16–18-day-old ratlings

	NAD	$NADH_2$	$NAD+$ $NADH_2$	$NAD/$ $NADH_2$	NADP	$NADPH_2$	$NADP+$ $NADPH_2$	$NADPH_2$ NADP
Normal	153 (8)	21 (4)	174	7·3	2·1 (8)	11·9 (8)	14·0	5·7
Dystrophic	170 (6)	27 (3)	197	6·3	1·7 (8)	8·0 (6)	9·7	4·7

Results are expressed as μg/g wet wt of retina. Number of estimations shown in parenthesis.

can be seen that no striking difference is apparent. It should be stressed, however, that these results are essentially preliminary, and that the difficulties inherent in the technique call for a much larger series of investigations. The present results are confined to an age group in which some initial imbalance might be expected. The method is at present being modified to produce greater accuracy and further studies are in progress.

REFERENCES

Berkow, J. W. and Patz, A. (1961a). *Arch. Ophthal.* **65**, 820.
Berkow, J. W. and Patz, A. (1961b). *Arch. Ophthal.* **65**, 828.
Cogan, D. C. and Kuwabara, T. (1959). *J. Histochem. Cyochem.* **7**, 334.
Cohen, L. and Noell, W. K. (1960). *J. Neurochem.* **5**, 253.
Dixon, M. and Webb, E. C. (1958). In *Enzymes*. Longmans, Green and Co., London.
Dumont, J. E. (1960). *Biochim. biophys. Acta* **40**, 354.
Futterman, S. (1963). *J. biol. Chem.* **238**, 1145.
Futterman, S. and Kinoshita, J. H. (1959a). *J. Biochem.* **234**, 723.
Futterman, S. and Kinoshita, J. H. (1959b). *J. Biochem.* **234**, 3174.
Graymore, C. N. (1964a), *Nature, Lond.* **201**, 615.
Graymore, C. N. (1964b), *Exp. Eye Res.* **3**, 5.
Graymore, C. N. (1960). *Br. J. Ophthal.* **44**, 363.
Graymore, C. N. and Towlson, M. (1965a). *Nature. Lond.* **206**, 1360.
Graymore, C. N. and Towlson, M. (1965b). *Vision Res.* **5**, 379.
Katz, J. and Wood H. G. (1960). *J. biol. Chem.* **235**, 2165.
Katz, J. and Wood H. G. (1963). *J. biol. Chem.* **238**, 517.
Kuwabara, T. and Cogan, D. C. (1959). *J. Histochem. Cytochem.* **7**, 334.
Kuwabara, T. and Cogan, D. C. (1960). *J. Histochem. Cytochem.* **8**, 214.

Lowry, O. H., Passonneau, J. V., Scultz, D. W. and Rock, M. K. (1961). *J. biol. Chem.* **236**, 2746.

Lowry, O. H., Roberts, N. H. and Lewis, C. (1956). *J. biol. Chem.* **220**, 879.

Rahman, M. A. and Kerly, M. (1961). *Biochem. J.* **78**, 536.

Slater, T. F., Heath, H. and Graymore, C. N. (1962). *Biochem. J.* **84**, 37P.

Slater, T. F. and Sawyer, B. (1962). *Nature, Lond.* **193**, 454.

DISCUSSION

PROFESSOR WALD commented on the dangers of high inbreeding inherent in the usual laboratory albino rat. His own personal experience had shown him that such colonies tended to develop their own particular characteristics, which not infrequently were appropriate to the investigations of the laboratory! His argument was that one tended to reject one's colony if it were unsuitable for the task in hand. This aspect should be considered when evaluating the most interesting results on the hypersensitivity of the rat visual cell to normal light reported by Professor Noell. He was very keen to hear more about this work, however, but thought it might well be worthwhile investigating strains from other laboratories. In replying to this comment, PROFESSOR NOELL stressed that he was only too aware of the problems of inbreeding, and that for this reason he had used three different strains of rats for his experiments on light sensitivity. All those he used showed the effect described, but he was not in a position to predict effects in lines not tested.

PROFESSOR WALD added that at one time he had equated the genetic abnormality of retinitis pigmentosa with some aberration of protein synthesis, most likely a failure to synthesise the protein moiety of rhodopsin in an adequate manner. It appeared, however, that in comparable congenital degenerative diseases in rats (Dowling and Sidman) opsin synthesis was increased, but he felt that this uncontrolled synthesis, of what he termed 'wild opsin' might well prove to have importance. As regards the suggestion that the rhodopsin of these animals might be abnormal, he reminded the meeting that the spectrum was quite normal. Nevertheless, this evidence did not invalidate the idea that there may be alterations in the non-chromophoric sites of the 'retinitis' rhodopsin, and this seemed to be a line well worth pursuing. The appropriate structure was probably required to permit rhodopsin molecules to fit into the quasi-crystalline structure of the outer segment.

He was particularly interested in Professor Noell's comment that there was an increase in metabolic activity around the time of cell death, but felt one had to be cautious in interpreting this. It might, for example, be analogous to the outpouring of insulin by the β-cells of the pancreas following destruction by alloxan, i.e., that this might be the moment of breakdown, in which release, as well as chaos, results. There was little reason to assume that this phenomenom was causative.

PROFESSOR WALD also stressed that the object of the pentose phosphate pathway was to provide hydrogens for reduction and synthesis—in this respect he felt the term alternative pathway should be abandoned as it inferred an alternative means of respiring. Far from yielding energy, this route utilized ATP and thus was in competition with other ATP requiring processes. This should be borne in mind when considering the effects of fluctuations in the activity of this pathway.

DR. READING thanked Professor Wald for his most useful comments, and agreed that the shunt mechanism should be regarded as a redox system providing electrons for reduction. His own belief was that the primary defect would be found to lie in some system coupled to the 'shunt' such as the lactic dehydrogenase or retinene reductase systems. Dr. Reading added that he was particularly interested in Professor Wald's comments regarding the synthesis of opsin, but felt that the scarcity of appropriate amounts of material prohibited this approach.

DR. CAMPBELL expressed pleasure at Dr. Newhouse's references during the meeting to her work demonstrating the possible importance of a defect in vitamin A metabolism in the aetiology of human retinitis pigmentosa. She showed the meeting a number of slides revealing marked improvement in the visual fields of patients under vitamin A therapy. There seemed little doubt that this helped inhibit the natural course of the disease (see *Symposium in Vitamin A Metabolism*, Exp. Eye Res. (1964)).

PROFESSOR COHEN commented generally on the obvious special vulnerability of the visual cell; it was evident from the papers presented in the session that many different factors were required for adequate maintenance of the delicately balanced visual cell. Professor Cohen suggested that the fact that degeneration occurs when function begins seemed to reflect some genetic inability to cope with the side effects of vision. The cones, for example, which presumably function to a lesser degree under normal light circumstances, are less susceptible.

In view of this, he felt that many diverse possibilities existed that might induce degeneration, such as release of retinene during bleaching, vitamin A deficiency, rhodopsin abnormalities, etc. His own prejudice led him to consider yet another line related to abnormalities of hydrogen ion concentration and distribution.

PROFESSOR BONAVITA commented on Professor Noell's reference to X-ray damage of the visual cells and reminded members that such treatment had been shown to speed up the progress of the developmental patterns of lactic acid dehydrogenase isoenzymes in the developing brain. This led in the rat treated by X-rays, to a pattern akin to that shown in the degenerate retina. As regards Dr. Graymore's estimations of pyridine nucleotides, he would like to say that they differed markedly from values found for the brain in his laboratory, in which the NAD/NADH ratio was very low. It was also of interest that in the developing brain, the change in this ratio had the opposite sign.

DR. KEEN asked DR. READING whether he had any information to suggest that changes in glycine incorporation were reflected by other amino acids. He also suggested that it might be of value to study the ultimate fate of amino acids using the technique of tissue autoradiography, as he felt that more information was required concerning the nature and distribution of the product protein.

DR. READING explained that he chose glycine as it was an amino acid that underwent little transamination. He had attempted autoradiography, but as yet had not perfected the technique. He added that so far there was no information on the abnormality of any specific protein in the degenerate retina.

In closing the discussion on the morning session, DR. COLE commented on the possibility that the extralamellar material of the degenerating retina might behave as a permeo-selective membrane favouring cation migration rather than anion migration. This would cause a greater change of potential for a given change of influx and would, for example, affect the c-wave of the ERG. He wondered whether some of the observed electrical changes might be accounted for in this way, as the result of altered ionic conductance, rather than of changes in active transport.

Notified Contribution to Discussion

Electrical Responses of the Eyes of Rats with Inherited Retinal Degeneration

G. B. Arden and Hisako Ikeda

Institute of Ophthalmology, University of London, England

In agreement with Dowling and Sidman (1962) it has been found that the waveform and the sensitivity of the electroretinogram (ERG) are normal up to the age of 18 days in rats with a hereditary retinal degeneration (Bourne, Campbell and Tansley, 1938). Subsequent to this, the ERG waveform alters, and the retinal sensitivity decreases. In young normal rats, with non-pigmented eyes, there is no c-wave, and there is no c-wave in the affected strain. The steady potential of the eye has been investigated, using the technique of induced eye movements. In normal rats, the amplitude of the steady potential increases with age. It reaches approximately 80% of the adult level by 20–25 days of age. The maturation is slower than that of the ERG, the rate of elongation of the outer limbs, or the rate of accumulation of rhodopsin. In the dystrophic rats, the normal increase of potential is observed in very young animals. However, at 20 days of age, a plateau is reached, and thereafter, the potential remains at about two-thirds the normal until about 60 days of age. It then drops rapidly to a low level. It is at this time that histological abnormalities of the pigment epithelium become obvious. This sequence is similar to the drop seen in experimental retinal detachment: a slight fall of potential occurs immediately after the detachment, but later, when the pigment epithelium atrophies, a profound fall of potential occurs (Ikeda and Foulds, 1964).

Light-induced changes in the steady potential can also be observed. They are related to the intensity of the adapting light, and reach an adult level more quickly than the absolute magnitude of the potential itself. In young dystrophic rats, aged less than 18 days, the light-induced changes are super-normal. This is the only electrophysiological correlate of biochemical overactivity which has been postulated in the developing abnormal retina (Noell, Bonavita, this Symposium). It occurs at a time when the ERG is quite normal, but extracellular rhodopsin-containing lamellae are accumulating rapidly.

After the 18th day, the light-induced change in the steady potential diminishes rapidly, so that by 20 days it is clearly subnormal. By 30–35 days, light adaptation causes no increase in the steady potential, and still later, causes a fall in potential.

The fact that the maturation of the light-induced change of potential is not the same as that of the steady potential *in toto* means that the experiments do not help in localizing the site of origin of the light-induced change. The fact that super-normality is observed at a time when the ERG is normal does not support the view that the production of the b-wave is closely related to the light-induced change. The similarity of the later changes with those observed in experimental retinal detachment lends support to the suggestion that the extracellular lamellar material acts as a barrier to retinal nutrition (Dowling and Sidman, 1962).

Details of this study will be published elsewhere.

REFERENCES

Bourne, M. C., Campbell, D. A. and Tansley, K. (1938). *Br. J. Ophthal.* **22**, 613.
Dowling, J. E. and Sidman, R. L. (1962). *J. Cell Biol.* **14**, 73.
Ikeda, H. and Foulds, W. S. (1964). *J. Physiol.* **172**, 36.

Some Aspects of Retinal Metabolism Revealed by Histochemistry

Müller Cells in the Pathological Condition*

Toichiro Kuwabara

Howe Laboratory of Ophthalmology, Massachusetts Eye and Ear Infirmary and Harvard Medical School, Boston, Mass., U.S.A.

In experimental damage of the retina the cellular reaction occurred first in the Müller cells characterized by swelling and migration of these cells. Instead of proliferating glial cells (including Müller cells), the reactive process of the retina seemed to be carried out by increasing the amount of glycogen and by maintaining high lactic acid dehydrogenase activity in the Müller cells.

1. Introduction

The importance of Müller cells as a nutritional supporting system of the retina has been emphasized in previous publications (Kuwabara, Cogan, Futterman and Kinoshita, 1959). Active dehydrogenase activity in the glycolytic pathway (Cogan and Kuwabara, 1959, Kuwabara and Cogan, 1960a), the storage and synthesis of glycogen (Kuwabara and Cogan, 1961; Hutchinson and Kuwabara, 1962) and the presence of other active enzymes (Lessell and Kuwabara, 1964) have been demonstrated histochemically in the Müller cells of various species.

Histological (Pedlar, 1962) and electron microscopic studies (Fine and Zimmerman, 1962) have revealed that the cytoplasmic processes of Müller cells are widely distributed throughout the entire thickness of the retina, except for the outer segments of the photoreceptors. Histological studies of the neuroglia of the retina (Lessell and Kuwabara, 1963) have shown that the number of other glial cells of the retina is relatively small and that the area occupied by Müller cells is incomparably larger than that of other glial cells.

Thus, Müller cells appear to be the most important glial elements of the retina. Presumably, Müller cells of the pathological retina also may play an important role in both metabolic and structural maintenance of the tissue.

The purpose of the present communication is to demonstrate how certain pathological conditions affect the metabolism of glycogen and the glycolytic enzymes of Müller cells.

2. Materials and Methods

Animal experiments

The animals used in these experiments were albino rabbits and cats having, respectively, partially vascularized and well-vascularized retinas. The retinas were damaged by a mechanical tear with a needle or the injection of a large amount of whole blood into the vitreous body. The animals were sacrificed at time intervals of 1 and 6 hr, 1 and 3 days, and 1, 4 and 10 weeks. At least 3 animals were used in each experiment.

Severe retinal damage was also induced by the systemic injection of a toxic dose of iodoacetic acid (20 mg/kg body weight, intravenously) and by the injection of a small

* This investigation was supported by U.S. Public Health Service Research grant NB–03015 from the National Institute of Neurological Diseases and Blindness, United States Public Health Service.

amount of 5% acetic acid into the vitreous body. The findings of these experiments will be reported in detail elsewhere.

Pieces of the freshly excised retina were incubated without sectioning in: (1) nitro blue tetrazolium solution in phosphate buffer at pH 7·8 with sodium lactate and NAD* (Kuwabara and Cogan, 1959) or (2) incubation media for glycogen synthesis (Kuwabara and Cogan, 1961). The former were fixed in formalin after an incubation of 30 min and sectioned in the frozen state; the latter were fixed in 95% alcohol after an incubation of 2 hr, and the paraffin sections were stained with PAS. The UDPG pathway was demonstrated in cryostat sections (Hutchinson and Kuwabara, 1962).

The rest of the tissue was divided into two pieces; one was fixed in formalin for general histological study and the other was fixed in alcohol for the demonstration of glycogen. Some representative eyes were specially fixed for electron microscopic study.

Clinicopathological material

Twenty-one eyes were obtained from the operating room of the Massachusetts Eye and Ear Infirmary: 16 eyes were enucleated for secondary glaucoma, 3 for melanomas, and 2 for injury of 2 months duration. One specimen of eviscerated material was obtained from an eye injured 1 week previously. Portions of all 22 retinas were treated according to one or the other of the methods described above. The vascular patterns of these retinas were studied by the trypsin digestion technique (Kuwabara and Cogan, 1960b).

3. Results

Animal experiments

Histology

Hemorrhagic or injected blood remained fluid inside the globe for 3–5 days. A clot was formed after about 7 days and absorption began within 3–4 weeks. The tissue in this experiment was obtained from the area adjacent to the tear or large blood coagulum. The severely damaged areas were usually studied histopathologically.

Swelling was the first response to the retinal damage. The swelling, shown as the wavy line of the external limiting membrane, occurred after 3 hr and continued for several days. By 6 hr the nuclei of Müller cells started to migrate into other layers, especially into the outer plexiform layer. Thickened fibers and hyperchromasia of both the nuclei and cytoplasm of Müller cells became conspicuous after 24 hr (Plate 1). The nuclei of some Müller cells often migrated as far as the outer nuclear layer and formed large pendulum-like bodies (Plate 2).

Electron microscopically, it was noted that the area occupied by Müller processes had increased considerably by 6 hr. This increase continued during the entire course of the experiment. The general micro-constituents of the cytoplasm did not differ greatly from the normal condition. However, an increased amount of rough surfaced endoplasmic reticulum was noted in several locations (Plate 3).

Müller cells at the border of severely damaged tissue did not show any different reaction from those in the general area. Severely damaged tissue usually disappeared within a short period of time without any trace of demarcation by the surrounding tissue. This punch-hole type response was most typified by the circumscribed necrotic tissue caused by acid coagulation.

The inflammatory cellular reaction was also curiously very small in these experimental conditions. Only a small number of infiltrating cells were noted in the vitreous or in the sub-retinal space. The choroid showed a more marked reaction.

---

*Abbreviations used: NAD, NADH, nicotinamide adenine dinucleotide and its reduced form, PAS, periodic acid-Schiff reaction; UDPG, uridine diphosphate glucose.

Glycogen

Glycogen was demonstrated by PAS staining with the accompanying control of salivary amylase digestion. The amount of native glycogen of the normal retina varied considerably according to the degree of vascularity of the retina. The results obtained from the rabbit and the cat will be presented separately.

Rabbit. The normally abundant glycogen of the Müller cells was found markedly reduced in amount during the period from 3 to 24 hr after the damage was induced in the retinas. The glycogen disappeared entirely from Müller cells in the necrotic retina and did not return during the period of investigation.

The surviving retinal tissue started to accumulate glycogen in the Müller cells after 2 days, and usually by 3 days the amount exceeded that of the normal retina. The glycogen was commonly seen as fine particles in the thickened Müller cells of the inner layers and in the bipolar cell layer, but often large bodies or droplets appeared extracellularly, formed, presumably, by coalescence of fine particles (Plate 4). This pathologically accumulated glycogen was relatively less soluble in water or in formalin than normal glycogen, although it was very sensitive to the amylase digestion.

Glycogen synthesis was observed to occur in direct relation to the amount of the stored glycogen. Synthetic glycogen was found strikingly in the outer half of Müller cells. The highest activity was seen after 3 days, and it continued for several weeks.

Cat. Except for the peripheral zone, normal cat retina contained very little glycogen. As long as the blood vessels were patent, the amount of glycogen in the Müller cells did not show any alteration. Cat retinas which had been damaged in a mild to moderate degree showed no excess glycogen, whereas retinas with severe vessel damage showed considerable accumulation of glycogen in their Müller cells. Glycogen synthesis also showed little alteration. It is noteworthy that glycogen synthesis by way of the UDPG pathway was most active in the outer nuclear layer of the retina.

Dehydrogenase activity

When the sensitive hydrogen acceptor, nitro blue tetrazolium, was used in the whole tissue incubation, it became almost impossible to eliminate non-specific background reactions. NADH diaphorase, which was distributed widely in the retinal tissue, especially in the mitochondria, was demonstrated by incubation with NAD. However, by the predominance in density and distribution of the formazan, the difference of the staining between the reactions induced by lactic acid-NAD and succinic acid was easily distinguishable. This distinction was more prominent when blue tetrazolium (BT) was used instead of nitro BT. The term "lactic acid dehydrogenase" in this communication, therefore, does not necessarily mean specific activity, and its histochemical coloration includes non-specifically induced NADH diaphorase activity.

Extremely high lactic acid dehydrogenase activity characterized normal Müller cells (Plate 5). The whole structural detail of the cell, including fine processes which extended into the complexity of the neuronal cells, was demonstrated by this enzyme staining.

The activity of lactic acid dehydrogenase in Müller cells seemed to be fairly constant in the pathological condition. The activity was not reduced even at early time periods after the damage, when all the glycogen was missing from the Müller cells. Heavy staining of the retina in the pathological condition by the lactic acid dehydrogenase system gave the impression that the activity in Müller cells had increased markedly

(Plate 6); but it appeared to be merely a quantitative increase due to the enlargement of the cytoplasmic material of Müller cells. The density of the formazan itself in the comparable areas of Müller cells between normal and pathological conditions did not show appreciable difference. The staining speed in the incubation media also was about the same. The overall heavy staining was observed in all pathological conditions as long as the Müller cells survived. Necrotic retina (in acid coagulation) or atrophic membranous retinal tissue did not stain.

Clinicopathological cases

Glaucoma

All 16 eyes showed similar chronic glaucomatous changes, including disappearance of the ganglion cells, thinning of the retinal tissue, hemorrhage, cystic change and occlusion of the vessels.

A marked increase in the glycogen content of the retina was noted in all cases. The glycogen deposition was seen throughout the entire thickness of the retina and was often concentrated in the bipolar cell layer where the glycogen synthesis, *in vitro*, was highest (Plate 7). The higher the glycogen deposition, the greater the amount of synthetic activity observed (Plate 8). (The native glycogen had been removed by amylase digestion before the incubation.) Heavy glycogen deposits were seen in the retinas in which the blood vessels were severely damaged. However, the totally atrophied thin retinal tissue did not contain any stored glycogen or show evidence of synthetic activity.

Enlarged Müller cells were stained with the lactic acid dehydrogenase system. Due to the increased cellular volume, in some cases the whole retinal tissue was diffusely stained dense blue (Plate 9).

Melanoma

Retinal tissue over the tumor and the peripheral area where the retinal tissue and the blood vessels had been damaged showed both a large amount of glycogen and high dehydrogenase activity. The retina away from the tumor mass did not differ from normal retina.

Injured detached retina

One case of necrotic retina from the excision and another from a disorganized hemorrhagic mass did not show any glycogen storage or dehydrogenase activity. The nuclear staining of the latter appeared to be normal, however.

Müller cells in another detached and disorganized retina showed about the same findings in glycogen metabolism and lactic acid dehydrogenase activity as in the cases of chronic glaucoma.

4. Comment

It was clear from these observations that the Müller cell was the first element of the retinal tissue to demonstrate reactions in pathological conditions. Before the response of the inflammatory cells occurred, the Müller cells swelled and their nuclei migrated. After the disappearance of the neuronal cells, the enlarged Müller cells occupied the space of the former cells. Although Müller cells did not show conspicuous proliferation or demarcation, they seemed to be the only reactive glial cells in the retina.

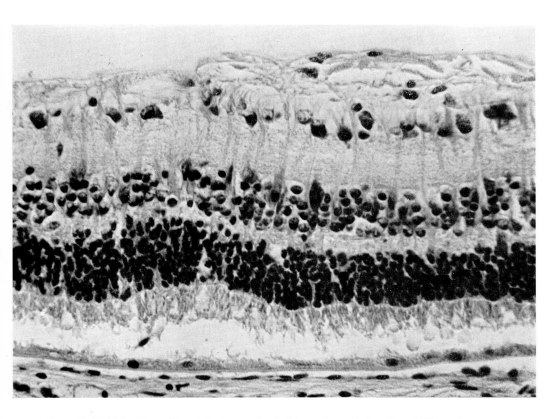

PLATE 1. Rabbit retina adjacent to the mechanical tear of 1-week-duration. Müller cells are conspicuous. Membranous tissue has formed on the inner limiting membrane. Hematoxylin and eosin. ($\times 256$)

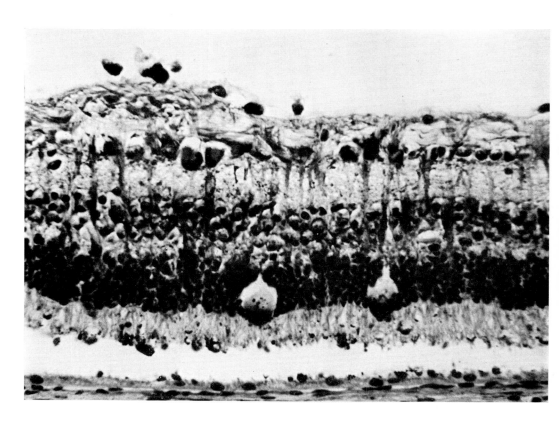

PLATE 2. Rabbit retina damaged by whole blood injection 1 week previously. Pendulum-like swelling of the Müller cells in the outer nuclear layer is seen. Some nuclei of the Müller cells have migrated into the outer plexiform layer. Large cells on the surface of the inner limiting membrane contain brown blood pigment granules. PAS. (×256)

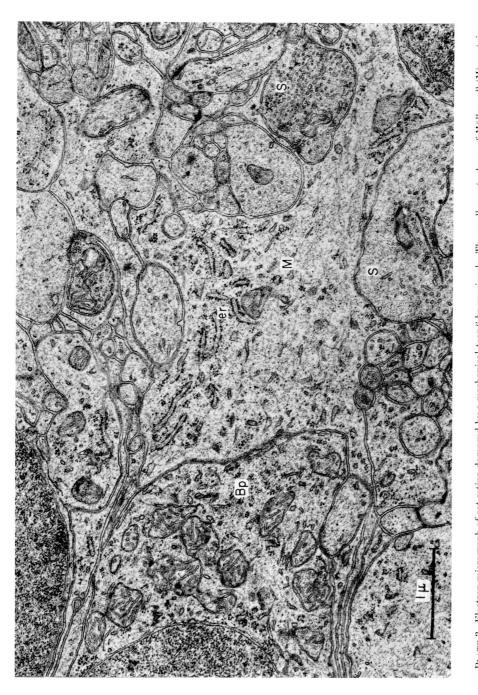

PLATE 3. Electron micrograph of cat retina damaged by a mechanical tear 6 hr previously. The swollen cytoplasm of Müller cell (M) contains an increased number of rough-surfaced endoplasmic reticulum (er). Bp: bipolar cell. S: cone-bipolar synapsis.

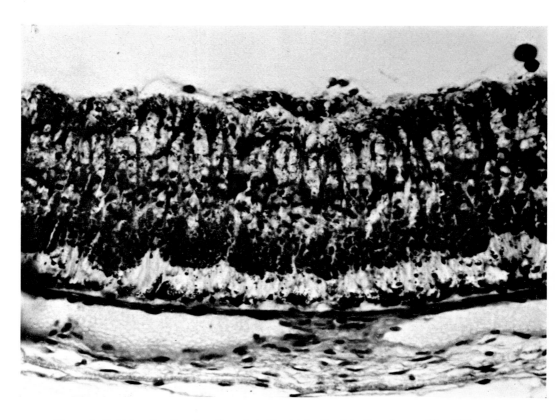

PLATE 4. Rabbit retina 7 weeks after whole blood injection into the vitreous. The Müller cells are enlarged and loaded with glycogen. PAS. (×256)

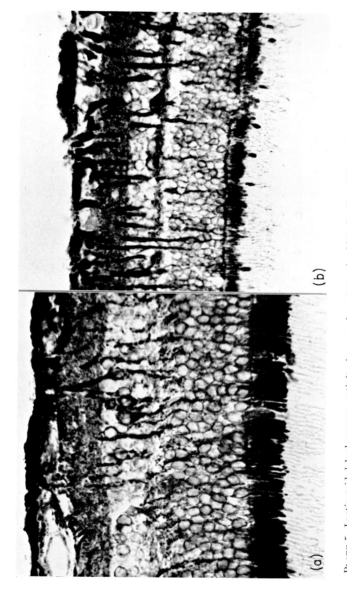

(a)

(b)

PLATE 5. Lactic acid dehydrogenase activity in normal cat (a) and rabbit (b). The Müller cells are delineated conspicuously by this enzyme stain. Heavy staining in the ellipsoid is due to non-specific NADH diaphorase activity. (×256)

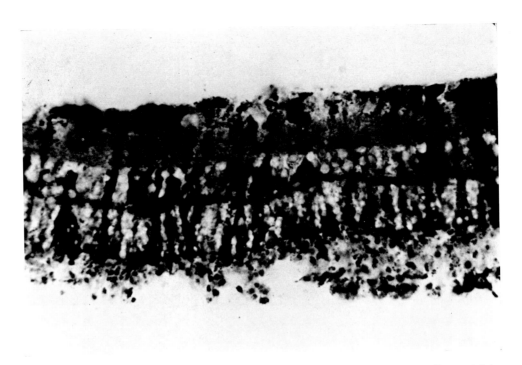

PLATE 6. Rabbit retina 3 weeks after the mechanical damage at the adjacent area. Dense staining of lactic acid dehydrogenase is seen in the swollen Müller cells. The photoreceptor area shows considerable damage. (×256)

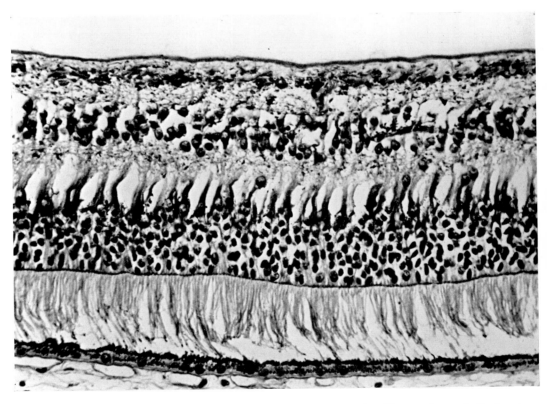

PLATE 7. Increased deposition of glycogen in the glaucomatous retina. Glycogen is seen in the inner layers and in the outer plexiform layer. PAS. (×256)

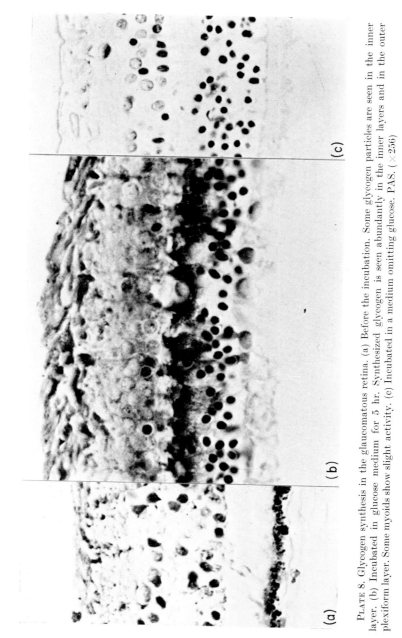

PLATE 8. Glycogen synthesis in the glaucomatous retina. (a) Before the incubation. Some glycogen particles are seen in the inner layer. (b) Incubated in glucose medium for 5 hr. Synthesized glycogen is seen abundantly in the inner layers and in the outer plexiform layer. Some myoids show slight activity. (c) Incubated in a medium omitting glucose. PAS. (×256)

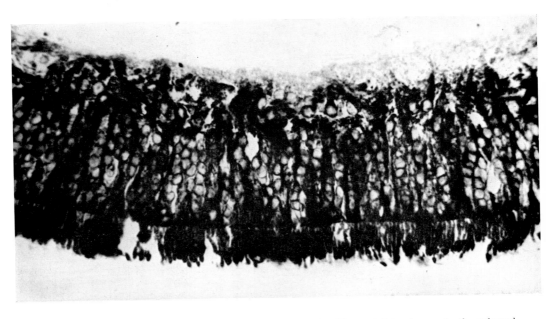

PLATE 9. Lactic acid dehydrogenase in glaucomatous retina. Dense staining is seen in the enlarged Müller cells. (×256)

It could not be denied that there was some increased cellularity in the inner layer of the "gliosed" retina; however, the number of these cells usually did not exceed that of the normal lemnocytes in the nerve fiber layer. The fibrous and gliosed appearance was thought to be dependent upon the enlargement of the Müller cells.

The disappearance of the stored glycogen from Müller cells, a short time after injury, might suggest that it was used in acute repair processes of the retina. Glycogen might have been stored for this purpose, especially in the non-vascularized retina. Müller cells in the damaged retina showed high synthetic activity of the glycogen and its storage. These were proportionally parallel to the vascular damage in the vascularized retina. It was interesting that this relationship was seen in the glycogen content of the normal retinas of various species: the amount being inversely proportional to the vascularity of the retina.

The typical proliferation of astrocytes and inflammatory infiltration which characterizes gliosis in the central nervous system did not occur in the retina. Instead, the preformed Müller cells showed increased anatomic and metabolic prominence. The cytoplasmic processes of the Müller cells ramified abundantly throughout the retina and the heightened metabolic activity of these cells expressed itself in increased glycogen synthesis and storage, increased diaphorase activity and increased ribosome content in the cytoplasm.

REFERENCES

Cogan, D. G. and Kuwabara, T. (1959). *J. Histochem. Cytochem.* **7**, 334.
Fine, B. S. and Zimmerman, L. E. (1962). *Invest. Ophthal.* **1**, 304.
Hutchinson, B. T. and Kuwabara, T. (1962). *Arch. Ophthal.* **68**, 538.
Kuwabara, T. and Cogan, D. G. (1959). *J. Histochem. Cytochem.* **7**, 329.
Kuwabara, T. and Cogan, D. G. (1960a). *J. Histochem. Cytochem.* **8**, 214.
Kuwabara, T. and Cogan, D. G. (1960b). *Arch. Ophthal.* **64**, 904.
Kuwabara, T. and Cogan, D. G. (1961). *Arch. Ophthal.* **66**, 680.
Kuwabara, T., Cogan, D. G., Futterman, S. and Kinoshita, J. H. (1959). *J. Histochem. Cytochem.* **7**, 67.
Lessell, S. and Kuwabara, T. (1963). *Arch. Ophthal.* **70**, 671.
Lessell, S. and Kuwabara, T. (1964). *Arch. Ophthal.* **71**, 851.
Pedler, C. (1962). *Documenta ophth.*, **16**, 208.

DISCUSSION

DR. KEEN referred to some discussion of the previous day relating to synthesis of glycogen by the retina. In view of the accepted difficulty of demonstrating insulin sensitivity of the whole retina, he was particularly anxious to ascertain whether inclusion of insulin in the incubating medium had any obvious effect on the metabolism of the Müller cells. DR. KUWABARA replied that from his own experience of experiments in which insulin had been omitted from the medium, he felt that the Müller cells were also insensitive.

PROFESSOR COHEN asked whether any information was available regarding the distribution of glucose-6-phosphatase in the retina. He thought that in terms of Dr. Kuwabara's findings it would be attractive to speculate that the glycogen of the Müller cells could supply glucose to the remainder of the retina, and that the high LDH activity might be concerned with gluco-neogenesis and replacing this glycogen.

He felt this type of system might have importance in Dr. Ames' system where recovery of function followed the initial loss in a low glucose medium (see Session 2). Perhaps, after an interval, the phosphatase system is activated and a normal level of glucose made available to the retina.

G

DR. KUWABARA said that glucose-6-phosphatase activity was localized in the inner layers and was related closely geographically to the sites of glycogen synthesis.

PROFESSOR WALD expressed great interest in the distinction in the extent of glycogen storage between the vascular and non-vascular retina. He recalled that some years ago he had observed that the isolated frog retina, without added substrate, remained active metabolically for many hours whereas that of the rat was entirely dependent on an added supply of glucose. Professor Wald also queried the statement that in the non-vascular retina all the glycogen was stored in the Müller cells. He wondered, therefore, what was the role of the paraboloid bodies, reputed to be composed of glycogen.

DR. KUWABARA explained that he had deliberately ignored these glycogen stores as they did not occur in the mammals to which he referred. He had looked at these bodies in lower animals and found them to behave in a similar way to the Müller cells, except that their ability to synthesize glycogen was less.

PROFESSOR NEWELL then emphasized a most important point when considering glycogen as an 'instant' energy source. Liver glycogen, he stressed, is a convenient source of glucose, but the glycogen of the eye, like that of muscle, is not mobilized in starvation. Although it is mobilized in hypoxia, this emergency supply of energy was called on only after all available supplies of glucose, ATP and phospho-creatine had been exhausted. A system such as this seemed to be rather inefficient, and he felt that one should not parallel this with that of the liver glycogen; the glycogen mobilized in hypoglycaemia may be of a very different type.

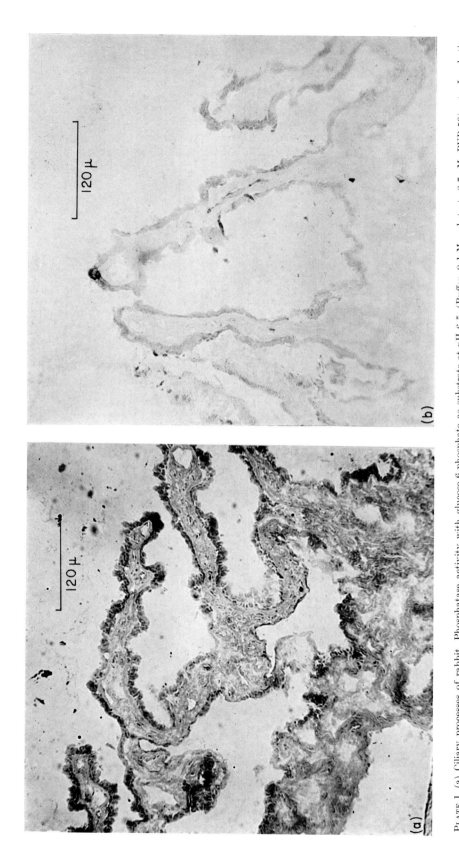

PLATE 1. (a) Ciliary processes of rabbit. Phosphatase activity with glucose-6-phosphate as substrate at pH 6·5. (Buffer, 0·1 M; substrate 6·7mM; PVP 5% w/v. Incubation 60 min counterstained eosin.) 5μ. (b) Sequential section to (a). Pre-incubated at pH 5·0 for 15 min at 37°C before incubating with glucose-6-phosphatase as (a).

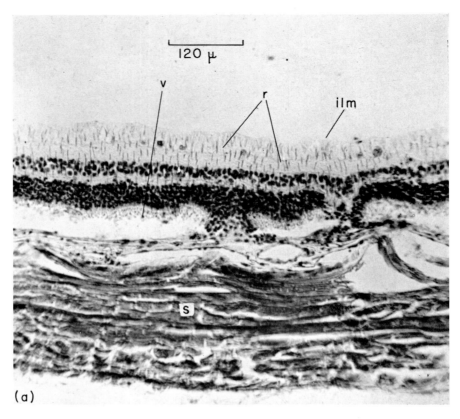

(a)

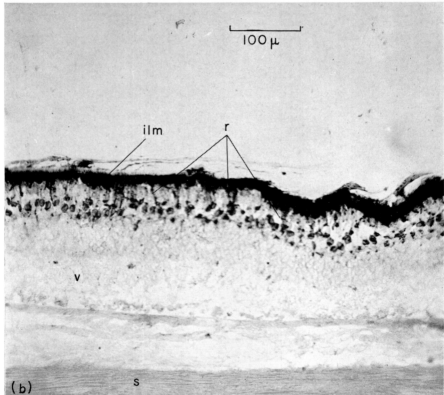

(b)

Plate 2. (a) Transverse section of rabbit retina, choroid and sclera. Mallory's PTAH after Biten-sky's formol-ethanol. 4μ. (b) Transverse section of retina (as (a)). Phosphatase activity with glucose-6-phosphate at pH 6·5. Counterstained with eosin. 4μ.
    ilm = inner limiting membrane; r = radial fibres; v = visual cell layer; s = sclera.

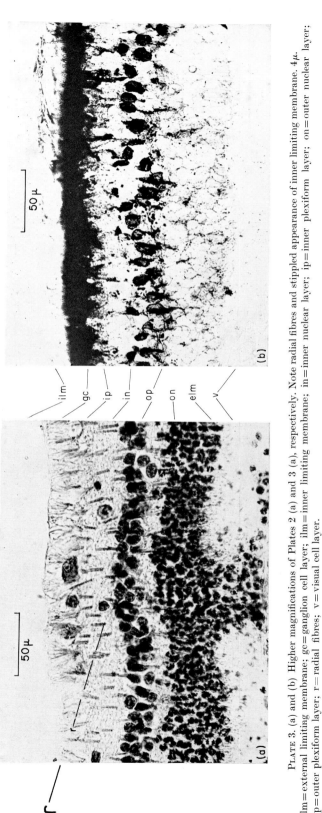

PLATE 3. (a) and (b) Higher magnifications of Plates 2 (a) and 3 (a), respectively. Note radial fibres and stippled appearance of inner limiting membrane. 4μ.
elm = external limiting membrane; gc = ganglion cell layer; ilm = inner limiting membrane; in = inner nuclear layer; ip = inner plexiform layer; on = outer nuclear layer; op = outer plexiform layer; r = radial fibres; v = visual cell layer.

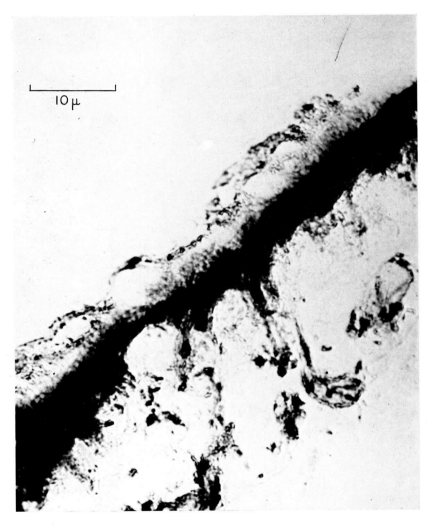

PLATE 4. High power of inner zone of rabbit retina. Phosphatase activity with glucose-6-phosphate at pH 6·5. Counterstained with eosin. 3μ.

Notified Contribution to Discussion
Glucose-6-Phosphatase in Ciliary Epithelium and Retina

Evan Cameron and D. F. Cole

Institute of Ophthalmology, University of London, England

What we have to say relates to a recent publication by Dr. Kuwabara on the distribution of phosphatases (Lessell and Kuwabara, 1964).

All our experiments have been conducted with tissues from albino rabbits.

During the course of experiments in which we were trying to demonstrate ouabain inhibition of a fraction of ATP-ase in ciliary epithelium (Cole, 1964) a number of other phosphate esters were used as substrates in the Wachstein and Meisel (1957) procedures in order to judge its specificity. Using glucose-6-phosphate there appeared to be much more phosphatase activity in the non-pigmented cell layer of the ciliary epithelium than in the pigment layer.

A separate study of glucose-6-phosphatase distribution has now been made, the enzyme being identified more narrowly by examining substrate specificity, pH optimum and inactivation at pH 5. In all these respects the material we refer to as glucose-6-phosphatase appeared to be identical with the glucose-6-phosphatase described by De Duve and associates (Beaufay and De Duve, 1954a,b; Beaufay, Hers, Berthet and De Duve, 1954; De Duve, Pressmann, Gianetto, Wattiaux and Appelmans, 1955) in the microsome fraction of centrifuged cells.

Apart from confirming our original idea about distribution in the ciliary epithelium sections of retina showed considerable glucose-6-phosphatase activity in the innermost segments of the Müller cells and possibly occasional bipolar cells.

According to the criteria of identification we have mentioned, our account of the localization of this enzyme confirms that of Dr. Kuwabara.

REFERENCES

Beaufay, H. and De Duve, C. (1954a). *Bull. Soc. Chim. biol.* **36**, 1525.
Beaufay, H. and De Duve, C. (1954b). *Bull. Soc. Chim. biol.* **36**, 1551
Beaufay, H., Hers, H. G., Berthet, J. and De Duve, C. (1954). *Bull. Soc. Chim. biol.* **36**, 1539.
Cole, D. F. (1964). *Exp. Eye Res.* **3**, 72.
De Duve, C., Pressmann, B. C; Gianetto, R; Wattiaux, R. and Appelmans, F. (1955). *Biochem. J.* **60**, 604.
Lessell, S., Kuwabara, T. (1964). *Arch. Ophthal.* **71**, 851.
Wachstein, M., Meisel, E. (1957). *Am. J. clin. Path.* **27**, 13.

Biochemical Mechanisms of Tetrazolium Salt Reduction

T. F. SLATER

Department of Chemical Pathology, University College Hospital Medical School, England

This communication briefly reviews the composition of several tetrazolium reductase systems present in rat liver suspensions and sections. The succinate-tetrazolium reductase systems of the mitochondrial fraction are considered in some detail as a main example. It is pointed out that, in such systems, the tetrazolium salt is reduced as an end reaction of a series of electron transfers involving varying segments of the respiratory chain. The fact that tetrazolium salts uncouple oxidative phosphorylation is discussed in terms of the linkage points of tetrazolium salts with the respiratory chain. Brief mention is made of the routes by which tetrazolium salts are reduced when coupled to the oxidation of reduced nicotinamide-adenine dinucleotides.

The need for caution in translating patterns of tetrazolium reduction into quantitative biochemical terms is stressed in view of the complexity of many tetrazolium reductase systems. The role of such artificial electron carriers as phenazine methosulphate in tetrazolium reductase systems is also discussed.

Reviews on the chemistry (Rust, 1955; Nineham, 1955) and biological applications (Cheronis and Stein, 1956; Novikoff, 1963; Pearse, 1960) of tetrazolium salts provide a comprehensive background to the topics discussed in this paper, which will be a brief review of certain aspects of tetrazolium reduction in tissue suspensions and tissue sections. The examples referred to will be taken largely from the author's own work and will illustrate a limited number of specific points. Although this meeting is specifically orientated towards the retina, no attempt will be made in this particular communication to consider the numerous papers concerning tetrazolium reduction in retinal preparations. Instead, the various difficulties which can arise in translating tetrazolium reduction *patterns* into quantitative *biochemical* terms, especially in so heterogeneous a tissue as the retina, will be considered. References to recent studies on tetrazolium reduction in retinal samples can be obtained from Kuwabara and Cogan (1960) and Nasu, Apponi and Viale (1962).

Among the first tetrazolium salts to be prepared was triphenyltetrazolium chloride (Von Pechmann and Runge, 1894). The structure is shown in Fig. 1 which also

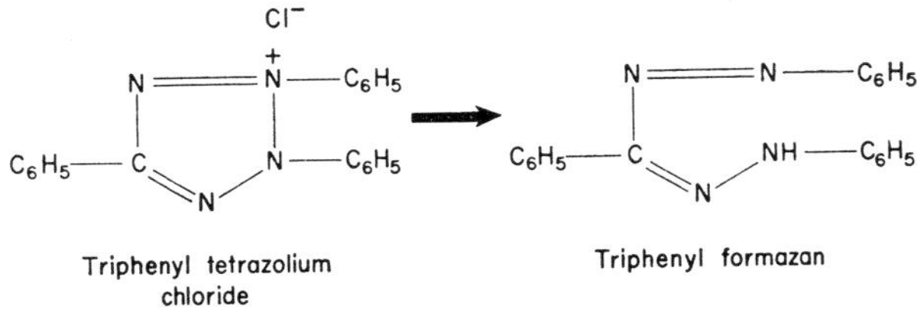

FIG. 1. Structural formulae of triphenyltetrazolium chloride and of triphenyl formazan.

illustrates that reduction of tetrazolium salts yields the formazans, the basis of their usefulness in biochemical and histochemical reactions.

A great variety of tetrazolium salts* have been described (e.g., see Nineham, 1955) but relatively few have been used (or found useful) in biology.

Tetrazolium salts can be reduced to the corresponding formazan by a variety of methods. At neutral pH strong reducing agents such as sodium dithionite or certain reduced quinones (Slater, 1959a; Lester and Ramasarma, 1959) will effect a rapid reaction. Weaker reductants such as vitamin C, reducing sugars and reducing steroids require alkaline conditions for a favourable reduction of tetrazolium salts to occur; some inorganic ions also reduce tetrazolium salts (Cheronis and Stein, 1956). Certain of these chemical methods of reduction have been utilized for the visualization of the particular reductant on chromatograms and on isoenzyme electrophoretograms (see Lederer and Lederer, 1953; Latner and Skillen, 1961).

Tetrazolium salts can also be reduced *via* interaction with certain enzyme systems of the oxido-reductase type. Since the end product of these reactions (formazan) is virtually insoluble in an aqueous medium, and thereby is deposited near the site of initial formation, such tetrazolium reactions have been used widely in histochemical demonstrations of dehydrogenase-linked systems in tissue sections (for a recent review see Barka and Anderson, 1963). Many investigators have measured the formazan produced in tissue sections and so have obtained quantitative measures of the level of enzyme activity (for example, Defendi and Pearson, 1955; Jardetsky and Glick, 1956). The quantitative approach has been critically assessed in a recent careful and detailed study (Jones, Maple, Aves, Chayen and Cunningham, 1963) and kinetic evaluation of tetrazolium reduction in such frozen sections now appears possible. Some use has also been made of tetrazolium reduction to quantitate enzyme-catalysed oxidations in tissue suspensions (e.g. Shelton and Rice, 1957; Sourkes and Lagnado, 1957; Kamin, Gibbs and Merritt, 1957; Slater and Planterose, 1960).

Since such enzyme sequences involve a dehydrogenase which functions in oxidizing the substrate, it was thought at first that tetrazolium salts were reduced *via* interactions with the dehydrogenase itself. However, in all instances where purified dehydrogenases have been used, no direct interaction with tetrazolium salts could be demonstrated (Shelton and Schneider, 1952; Farber, Sternberg and Dunlop, 1956; Nachlas, Margulies and Seligman, 1960; Lester and Smith, 1961). Additional electron carriers have to be present to mediate between the dehydrogenase and the tetrazolium salt thereby making the system relatively complex in nature. Such carriers can be the natural components of a complex enzyme sequence (e.g., the components of the respiratory chain) or they can be added artificially (e.g., phenazine methosulphate and vitamin K_3).

As already mentioned, it is the purpose of this communication to review briefly the evidence available as to the composition of representative enzyme systems which can be coupled to the reduction of tetrazolium salts. The first example which will illustrate the complexity of some such systems will concern the nature of the rat liver enzyme system which couples succinate oxidation to tetrazolium reductions; and only the results obtained with one tetrazolium salt, neotetrazolium chloride,† will be men-

---

* Abbreviations used: TTC, triphenyltetrazolium chloride; INT, 2-p-nitrophenyl-3-p-iodophenyl-5-phenyl tetrazolium chloride; NT, 2, 2′, 5, 5′-tetraphenyl-3, 3′-(p-diphenylene) ditetrazolium chloride; NBT, 2, 2′-di-p-nitrophenyl-5, 5′-diphenyl-3, 3′ (3, 3′-dimethoxy-4, 4′-diphenylene) ditetrazolium chloride; MTT, C, N-diphenyl-N′-4, 5-dimethyl thiazol-2-yl tetrazolium bromide.

† The samples of neotetrazolium chloride used in the studies reported by the author were recrystallized from commercial samples. It is probable (see Okui, Suzuki, Momose and Ogamo, 1963) that such material consisted of a mixture of neotetrazolium chloride and 2, 5-diphenyl-3-diphenylenetetrazolium chloride. In this article, therefore, 'NT' must be considered to represent the above mixture.

tioned in any detail. The nomenclature used will follow the suggestions of the *International Union of Biochemistry, Report of the Commission on Enzymes* (1961). For example, the enzyme systems coupling succinate oxidation with tetrazolium reduction are described as succinate-tetrazolium reductase systems. The generic term succinate-tetrazolium reductase will be used when remarks are general in character and can be applied to tetrazolium results as a whole; when the remarks are intended to apply to a particular tetrazolium salt, the enzyme system will be described more specifically, for instance, succinate-neotetrazolium reductase system.

Succinate is oxidized in the mitochondrial fraction of rat liver (and many other tissues) by interaction with succinate dehydrogenase. This flavoprotein enzyme is coupled in an orientated fashion with a sequence of cytochromes and other substances which together constitute the respiratory chain. The finer details of this complex structure are still not known but the arrangement (Fig. 2) is thought to represent in a

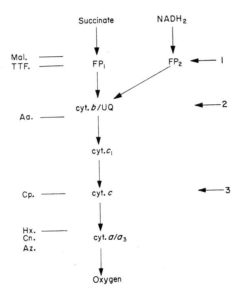

FIG. 2. Diagram of the rat-liver respiratory chain used for the purposes of this communication. FP_1 and FP_2 represent the dehydrogenase flavoproteins. Cytochrome is abbreviated cyt. and ubiquinone is abbreviated to UQ in the figure. The three arrows (1, 2, 3) indicate regions at which oxidative phosphorylation is thought to occur (see Slater, 1958). The points on the respiratory chain at which the inhibitors mentioned in the text are taken to exert their effects are shown on the left-hand side of the respiratory chain components. Malonate, Mal; thenoyltrifluoroacetone, TTF; antimycin A, Aa; chlorpromazine, Cp; hydroxylamine, Hx; cyanide, Cn; azide, Az.

general fashion the main oxidation-reduction framework involved (for recent reviews dealing with this point see Massey and Veeger, 1963; Ernster and Lee, 1964). Figure 2 also indicates the corresponding pathway by which $NADH_2$ is oxidized in mitochondrial fractions, and the 3 positions on the respiratory chain at which oxidative phosphorylation is known to occur (for references, see Slater, 1958; Lehninger and Wadkins, 1962).

If rat liver mitochondria are incubated aerobically with succinate and a suitable buffer system, oxygen is utilized and succinate is oxidized to fumarate. The addition of NT to such a system diverts part of the electron flow from oxygen towards the production of formazan. In commonly accepted nomenclature, NT has been reduced by the succinate-NT reductase system. Since succinate is itself oxidized by interaction with a series of electron transferring components (see Fig. 2) the question as to the mechanism of NT reduction (i.e., with which component does it interact?) can be seen to have no simple or immediate answer.

As mentioned earlier, it has been shown that none of the tetrazolium salts so far tested will couple directly with purified dehydrogenases; this includes succinate dehydrogenase. Thus, the reduction of tetrazolium salts coupled to succinate oxidation occurs via an interaction further along the respiratory chain than the primary dehydrogenase. Considerable efforts have been made to evaluate the precise point(s) and in such work the use of metabolic inhibitors has played a vital role. Many inhibitors are now known which block specific regions of the respiratory chain thus stopping electron flow in the regions distal to the point of action (in this context 'distal' means nearer oxygen). Thus, by studying the effects of such inhibitors on tetrazolium reduction it is possible to gain considerable information concerning the site of interaction of the tetrazolium salt with the respiratory chain. The points of action of the major inhibitors used in such 'chemical dissection' are also shown in Fig. 2 (see Green, 1961). The following remarks, taken largely from Slater (1959b, 1963) unless otherwise stated, will illustrate the method of approach as applied to NT. The levels of inhibitors used were those known to be effective in blocking electron transport along the respiratory chain.

Succinate-NT reductase is strongly inhibited by malonate, thenoyltrifluoroacetone and antimycin A. These results indicate that under aerobic conditions approximately 90% of the reduction occurs via an interaction distal to the antimycin A sensitive region, believed to be at the level of the reoxidation of reduced ubiquinone (Pumphrey and Redfearn, 1959; Green, Hatefi and Fechnier, 1959; also see Szarkowska and Klingenberg, 1963). The remaining 10% of the reduction could, on the basis of the components shown in Fig. 2, occur via an interaction of NT with reduced cytochrome b or reduced ubiquinone. Since some reduced quinones interact rapidly with tetrazolium salts (Slater, 1959a; Lester and Ramasarma, 1959) the latter interaction has been the more favoured (Slater, 1963).

In view of the probable occurrence of other tetrazolium salts in commercial samples of 'NT', it is possible that the 10% reduction which is insensitive to antimycin A results from one of these extra components.

The major part of NT reduction in rat liver mitochondria under aerobic conditions, however, occurs via an interaction between cytochrome c_1 and oxygen. 'Chlorpromazine' inhibits the succinate-neotetrazolium reductase reaction to a similar extent to its effect on oxygen uptake; its point of respiratory inhibition has been suggested to be through a competition with cytochrome c (Dawkins, Judah and Rees, 1959). Inhibitors of cytochrome oxidase have little effect on the succinate-NT reductase system, implying that the interaction of NT with the respiratory chain is not through this complex. Thus, NT appears to be mainly reduced via an interaction at the level of cytochrome c. However, neither reduced cytochrome c_1, nor reduced cytochrome c, will directly reduce NT (Lester and Smith, 1961) indicating that some additional factor is involved. This had previously been inferred by an analysis of the so-called 'non-linear response' of the succinate-neotetrazolium reductase system (Slater, 1959b).

The above remarks are summarized in Fig. 3 which also includes results obtained with other tetrazolium salts to be mentioned later. One further fact may be mentioned to add to the complexity of the neotetrazolium system. The overall rate of formazan production is affected by the partial pressure of oxygen in the incubation medium (Slater, 1963). Anaerobic conditions stimulate the reduction of NT but the increase is not proportionately equal at the two sites. The early antimycin A insensitive site is stimulated much more by anaerobic conditions and, in fact, then becomes of equal importance with the reaction occurring at the level of cytochrome c.

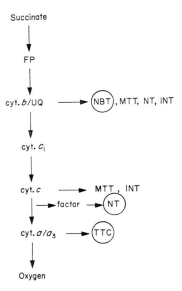

FIG. 3. The postulated points of interaction of the tetrazolium salts mentioned in the text. The major site of reduction under aerobic condition is in each case shown encircled. For abbreviations see text.

Thus, the succinate-NT reductase system is a complex sequence of components and the reduction of NT involves at least two interactions, the relative proportions of which may change under certain conditions of anoxia. It is self-evident that a change in the concentration or 'efficiency' of any components of the system, sufficient to affect the overall activity of the respiratory chain, will affect the kinetics of the succinate-NT reductase system.

Similar studies on succinate-NT reductase systems in suspensions of a variety of tissues have recently been made by other investigators (Nachlas et al., 1960; Lester and Smith, 1961; Oda and Okazaki, 1958; Miura, Aso, Mashima and Nagata, 1962). All agree that the system is complex although, understandably, there is some divergence of opinion as to the relative importance of the sites of reduction. These differences are probably due to different assay conditions and differences in experimental material and inhibitor concentrations. Variations in the purity of tetrazolium samples are probably significant in this connection (see Burtner, Bahn and Longley, 1957; Okui et al., 1963; also footnote on p. 101. It is desirable that the major points reported in previous communications, based on work with commercial samples of tetrazolium salts, should be checked using samples purified by chromatographic procedures. Until this is done, both histochemical and biochemical results obtained with commercial samples should be recognized as possibly representing in each case the reduction of mixtures of tetrazolium salts.

Similar investigations to those described above for NT with tissue suspensions have been reported using other tetrazolium salts (Nachlas et al., 1960; Lester and

Smith, 1961; Slater, Sawyer and Strauli, 1963). Evidence leading to the following conclusion will not be discussed here: briefly, the composition of each succinate-tetrazolium reductase system studied was found to be complex in character and to involve varying segments of the respiratory chain. For example, in rat liver suspensions under aerobic conditions, NBT couples mainly at the level of ubiquinone, whereas TTC reacts mainly with cytochrome oxidase (Slater et al., 1963). These conclusions are also summarized in Fig. 3.

The studies described so far were all performed with tissue or mitochondrial suspensions yet it is with tissue sections that tetrazolium salts are most used and most useful. A recent study (Slater and Smith, 1964) has been concerned with evaluating the similarities and differences between succinate-tetrazolium reductases in suspensions and in 6 μ-thick frozen sections of rat liver. Two tetrazolium salts have so far been investigated, NBT and MTT, and the general conclusions reached with sections were identical with those previously described for rat liver homogenates (Slater et al., 1963; Slater and Smith, 1964). There are several other indications in the literature that tetrazolium salts are reduced by similar pathways in sections as in suspensions (see, for example, Farber et al., 1956; Cogan and Kuwabara, 1959; Jardetsky and Glick, 1956; Pearse, 1960). From such work it seems reasonable to conclude that the reduction of tetrazolium salts in tissue sections proceeds via complex sequences of interactions (as found in suspensions) involving widely differing components. Interpretation of tetrazolium reduction patterns must, as a consequence, be made in the light of such information concerning the composition of the reacting system. The final reduction of the tetrazolium salt can be seen to be the terminal and virtually irreversible stage in a sequence of electron transfers, any one of which, under abnormal conditions, could conceivably become rate-limiting and thereby govern the overall kinetics of the system.

Although purified succinate dehydrogenase does not react with any of the tetrazolium salts so far tried, suitable electron carriers can mediate and promote electron transfer from the dehydrogenase direct to a variety of tetrazolium salts. For example, phenazine methosulphate can function in this manner (Farber and Bueding, 1956; Nachlas et al., 1960). Methylene blue (Zollner and Rothermund, 1954) and vitamin K$_3$ (Slater, 1959b) behave in a similar fashion in mitochondrial suspensions although with these compounds the interaction may not be with the primary dehydrogenase as is known to be the case with phenazine methosulphate (see Singer, Kearney and Massey, 1957). Thus, in tissue samples supplemented with an electron carrier such as phenazine methosulphate, the sequential composition of the various succinate-tetrazolium reductase systems is altered in favour of (biochemically) a less complex sequence. Since reduced phenazine methosulphate reduces tetrazolium salts directly and non-enzymically, it can be seen that the only enzyme process in such a supplemented system is the primary succinate dehydrogenase itself. It might be thought, therefore, that such a simplification has much to commend it in histochemical terms but the commendations are biochemical in nature and histochemical evaluation of such a system involves very different criteria.

The systems coupling the oxidation of reduced nicotinamide-adenine dinucleotide (NADH$_2$) to tetrazolium reduction in rat liver mitochondria have not been studied in such detail as the succinate-tetrazolium reductase systems (see Slater, 1959c; Lester and Smith, 1961). In the case of NT it is known that the reductase system is insensitive to Amytal (Slater, 1959c) and the coupling site could conceivably be via the NADH$_2$-flavoprotein or the lipoyl dehydrogenase reaction (Massey, 1960). If part at least of the reaction proceeds through the first pathway then it can be seen that NT reacts with the respiratory chain at three points: at the levels of ubiquinone and cytochrome c (with succinate as substrate) and at the level of $NADH_2$-flavoprotein ($NADH_2$ as substrate). These regions are suggestively close to the loci of oxidative phosphorylation (see Slater, 1958; but see also Ramirez and Mujica, 1964; Smith and Hansen, 1964). Thus, the possibility arises that part at least of tetrazolium reduction coupled to succinate- or $NADH_2$-oxidation is through an interaction with components of the side-chain phosphorylation sequences and not with the respiratory chain members themselves. Such interactions could explain the failure to obtain direct coupling between reduced respiratory chain components (such as cytochromes c_1 and c) and tetrazolium salts. Evidence supporting this proposal (Slater, 1963) has recently been obtained by the demonstration that all tetrazolium salts tested uncoupled phosphorylation in rat liver mitochondria at low final concentration (for example, 18 μM for NT; Clark, Slater and Greenbaum, 1964).

An objection to such a route for tetrazolium reduction being the major one is that most work on tetrazolium reductase systems has been with tissue samples in a non-phosphorylating condition. However, it is possible that although the overall oxidative phosphorylation system is non-functional, tetrazolium salts could still accept electrons from an early stage of the process. Interaction at an early stage could explain the lack of inhibition on succinate-tetrazolium reductase systems displayed by dicoumerol at concentrations known to uncouple phosphorylation (Cooper and Lehninger, 1956). Dicoumerol only inhibited tetrazolium reduction at a very high 'concentration' and when in suspension form (Slater, 1963). On the other hand, dinitrophenol partially inhibits the succinate-neotetrazolium reductase system (Slater, 1963).

Although the compositions of the sequence(s) concerned in oxidative phosphorylation are not yet fully established (for a recent review see Lehninger and Wadkins, 1962) several reports have suggested a role for quinones in the overall reaction (e.g., Beyer, 1959). Several chemical schemes for phosphorylation have been drawn up using quinol-phosphates as intermediates (Chmielewska, 1960; Clark and Todd, 1960). Such indications of quinone-like substances in the phosphorylation reactions are of interest to tetrazolium reduction since several reduced quinones will interact rapidly and non-enzymically with tetrazolium salts (Slater, 1959a; Lester and Ramasarma, 1959; Tranzer and Pearse, 1963).

From such considerations it can be realized that succinate- and $NADH_2$-tetrazolium reductase systems are complex in nature. The final reduction follows a series of electron transfers culminating in the virtually irreversible precipitation of the formazan. At present, little is known of the rate-determining stages in such reactions so that it can be seen to be unwise to label such systems in terms of the primary dehydrogenase alone, without careful investigation, since this infers not only that the system is simple in character but that the overall rate of reaction bears a direct relationship to the activity of the dehydrogenase. This must not be construed to mean that results of considerable importance cannot be obtained by studies with tetrazolium reductase systems, but only that the results should not be interpreted in too simple or unequivocal a manner in the absence of adequate data.

Turning now very briefly to other types (e.g., extra-mitochondrial) of tetrazolium reductase system we shall find that these also do not involve simple dehydrogenase-tetrazolium salt interactions. Further, in several cases, the overall complexity of the system can result in the final formazan deposition appearing in a different intracellular site from that of the primary dehydrogenase in the sequence. This effect is best illustrated by an example. In normal liver, lactic dehydrogenase is mainly a soluble enzyme using the standard criteria of differential centrifuging (Novikoff, 1963). However, in tissue sections, formazan produced as a result of lactate metabolism is deposited on (or in) the mitochondria. This apparent discrepancy between two methods of approach is readily resolved when the composition of the lactate-tetrazolium reductase system is examined. Lactic dehydrogenase itself (like glucose-6-phosphate dehydrogenase, Slater, unpublished results) does not react directly with tetrazolium salts. Further, the $NADH_2$ formed as a result of lactate oxidation cannot itself reduce tetrazolium salts (Slater, 1959). The actual production of formazan results from an interaction with a $NADH_2$ oxidase system which, in rat liver, is largely mitochondrial in localization. As previously mentioned, tetrazolium salts can interact with such $NADH_2$-oxidase systems and, as a consequence, the formazan is precipitated largely in the mitochondria. Such conclusions have been strongly stressed on previous occasions by several authors (Novikoff, 1963; Kuwabara and Cogan, 1960; Farber et al., 1956).

Thus, we see that the discrepancy between centrifugation analysis and tetrazolium staining in tissue sections is due to the inclusion in the tetrazolium system of an extra sequence of steps, necessary for the overall reaction, and yet differing in intracellular localization from the initial dehydrogenase which it was hoped to visualize.

Not only must interpretations as to the intracellular *localization* of dehydrogenases visualized by tetrazolium methods be viewed cautiously in the light of the foregoing remarks, but impressions of the *level* of dehydrogenase activity can also be misleading. For instance, in the sequence shown in Fig. 4 either enzyme step (or even the non-

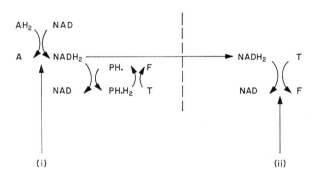

(i)   (ii)

Fig. 4. A schematic representation of the sequence of events coupling the oxidation of a substrate by a dehydrogenase in an extra-mitochondrial region of a liver cell with tetrazolium reduction through a $NADH_2$-tetrazolium reductase in the mitochondrial fraction. The dehydrogenase is depicted to act at point (i) and the $NADH_2$-tetrazolium reductase at point (ii). The coupling of $NADH_2$ with phenazine methosulphate (PH) and consequent reduction of tetrazolium (T) to formazan (F) is also shown. The vertical dashed line represents the phase barrier between the dehydrogenase in the soluble fraction and the $NADH_2$-tetrazolium reductase in the mitochondrial fraction of the cell.

enzymic steps) may be rate-limiting. Only in the case of reaction (i) being clearly rate-limiting will variations in formazan production have any relevance to the activity of the primary dehydrogenase. Although this has been reported to be generally the case for many $NADH_2$-linked reactions coupled to tetrazolium reduction (Barka and Anderson, 1963), in frozen sections of rat liver Jones and McCabe (pers. comm.) have found that with lactate or β-hydroxybutyrate as substrate the rate-determining stage is at the level of the $NADH_2$-tetrazolium reductase.

It is in difficult situations like those mentioned above that the addition of phenazine to the reaction mixture could give valuable information concerning the activity of the primary dehydrogenase. As shown in Fig. 4 phenazine can accept directly from $NADH_2$ and donate directly to tetrazolium salts. Thus, the system involves only one enzymic step—the primary dehydrogenase. Although the picture obtained in the presence of phenazine may be less satisfactory, histochemically speaking, the amount of formazan deposition would be a better reflection of changes in primary dehydrogenase activity. Further experiments performed with phenazine methosulphate might show up dehydrogenase activity in regions of a heterogenous tissue (e.g., retina) where previously none was imagined present due to the lack of appreciable $NADH_2$- or $NADPH_2$-tetrazolium reductase systems at those sites.

Only very brief mention will be made of NADP-linked reactions and only to raise a cautionary note. In histochemical studies in which the final deposition of formazan occurs at the site of $NAD(P)H_2$-tetrazolium reductase activity, the intracellular site may be confused by the occurrence of high NAD-NADP transhydrogenase reactions. Thus, to quote a hypothetical example, if the primary dehydrogenase is NADP-linked and high transhydrogenase activity is present, the final formazan deposit will reflect not only the site of $NADPH_2$-tetrazolium reductase activity but also that of the $NADH_2$-system which may have a different localization.

This communication has attempted to point out the general features of several kinds of tetrazolium reductase system. Much emphasis has been laid on the complex nature of such systems and of the caution required in interpreting the results in biochemical terms. However, it is hoped that such caution and criticism as have been raised will prove of a constructive rather than of a destructive form, since it is felt that tetrazolium staining reactions have much to contribute in the justified expansion of histochemical procedures.

ACKNOWLEDGMENTS

I am grateful to Mrs. B. Sawyer and Miss U. D. Strauli for assistance, and to the Agricultural Research Council for a grant making such assistance possible.

REFERENCES

Barka, T. and Anderson, P. J. (1963). In *Histochemistry, Theory, Practice and Bibliography*. Hoeber Medical Division, Harper and Row, London.
Beyer, R. E. (1959). *J. biol. Chem.* **234**, 688.
Burtner, H. J., Bahn, R. C. and Longley, J. B. (1957). *J. Histochem. Cytochem.* **5**, 127.
Cheronis, N. D. and Stein, H. (1956). *J. Chem. Educ.* **33**, 120.
Chmielewska, J. (1960). *Biochim. biophys. Acta* **39**, 170.
Clark, V. M. and Todd, A. R. (1960). In *Quinones in Electron Transport*, CIBA Foundation Symposium. Churchill, London.
Clark, J., Slater, T. F. and Greenbaum, A. L. (1965). *Biochem. J.* **94**, 651.
Cogan, D. G. and Kuwabara, T. (1959). *J. Histochem. Cytochem.* **7**, 334.
Cooper, L. and Lehninger, A. L. (1956). *J. biol. Chem.* **219**, 519.
Dawkins, M. J. R., Judah, J. D. and Rees, K. R. (1959). *Biochem. J.* **72**, 204.
Defendi, V. and Pearson, B. (1955). *J. Histochem. Cytochem.* **3**, 61.
Ernster, L. and Lee, C. (1964). In *Annual Reviews of Biochemistry*, p. 729. Annual Reviews Inc., Palo Alto.
Farber, E. and Bueding, E. (1956). *J. Histochem. Cytochem.* **4**, 357.
Farber, E., Sternberg, W. H. and Dunlap, C. E. (1956). *J. Histochem. Cytochem.* **4**, 284.
Green, D. E. (1961). *5th International Congress Biochemistry*. Plenary Lecture, Moscow.
Green, D. E., Hatefi, Y. and Fechnier, W. F. (1959). *Biochem. biophys. Res. Comm.* **1**, 45.
Jardetsky, C. D. and Glick, D. (1956). *J. biol. Chem.* **218**, 283.

Jones, G. R. N., Maple, A. J., Aves, E. K., Chayan, J. and Cunningham, G. J. (1963). *Nature, Lond.* **197**, 568.

Kamin, H., Gibbs, R. H. and Merritt, A. D. (1957). *Fed. Proc.* **16**, 202.

Kuwabara, T. and Cogan, D. G. (1960). *J. Histochem. Cytochem.* **8**, 214.

Latner, A. L. and Skillen, A. W. (1961). *Lancet* (ii), 1286.

Lederer, E. and Lederer, M. (1953). *Chromatography.* Elsevier, Amsterdam.

Lehninger, A. L. and Wadkins, C. L. (1962). In *Annual Reviews of Biochemistry*, p. 47. Annual Reviews, Inc., Palo Alto.

Lester, R. L. and Ramasarma, E. M. (1959). *J. biol. Chem.* **234**, 672.

Lester, R. L. and Smith, A. (1961). *Biochim. biophys. Acta* **47**, 475.

Massey, V. (1960). *Biochim. biophys. Acta* **37**, 314.

Massey, V. and Veeger, C. (1963). In *Annual Reviews of Biochemistry*, p. 579. Annual Reviews Inc., Palo Alto.

Miura, Y., Aso, Y., Mashima, Y. and Nagata, I. (1962). *J. Biochem. Tokyo* **52**, 43.

Nachlas, M. M., Margulies, S. I. and Seligman, A. M. (1960). *J. biol. Chem.* **235**, 2739.

Nasu, H., Apponi, G. and Viale, G. L. (1962). *Z. fur Zellforsch.* **56**, 188.

Nineham, A. W. (1955). *Chem. Rev.* **55**, 355.

Novikoff, A. B. (1963). In *Histochemistry and Cytochemistry*, Proceedings of 1st Int. Congr., Paris, 1960, ed. R. Wegmann, Pergamon Press, London.

Oda, T. and Okasaki, H. (1958). *Acta Med. Okayama.* **12**, 193.

Okui, S., Suzuki, Y., Momose, K. and Ogamo, A. (1963). *J. Biochem. Tokyo* **53**, 500.

Pearse, A. G. E. (1960). In *Histochemistry, Theoretical and Applied.* Churchill, London.

Pumphrey, A. and Redfearn, E. R. (1959). *Biochem. J.* **72**, 2P.

Ramirez, J. and Mujica, A. (1964). *Biochim. biophys. Acta* **86**, 1.

Rust, J. B. (1955). *Trans. N.Y. Acad. Sci.* **17**, 379.

Shelton, E. and Schneider, W. C. (1952). *Anat. Rec.* **112**, 61.

Shelton, E. and Rice, M. E. (1957). *J. natn. Cancer Inst.* **18**, 117.

Singer, T. P., Kearney, E. B. and Massey, V. (1957). *Adv. Enzymol.* **18**, 65.

Slater, E. C. (1958). *Adv. Enzymol.* **20**, 147.

Slater, T. F. (1959a). *Nature, Lond.* **183**, 50.

Slater, T. F. (1959b). *Biochem. J.* **73**, 314.

Slater, T. F. (1959c). *Nature, Lond.* **183**, 1679.

Slater, T. F. (1963). *Biochim. biophys. Acta* **77**, 365.

Slater, T. F. and Planterose, D. N. (1960). *Biochem. J.* **74**, 591.

Slater, T. F., Sawyer, B. C. and Strauli, U. D. (1963). *Biochim. biophys. Acta* **77**, 383.

Slater, T. F. and Smith, J. F. (1964). *Biochim. biophys. Acta* in press.

Smith, A. L. and Hansen, M. (1964). *Biochem. biophys. Res. Comm.* **15**, 431.

Sourkes, T. L. and Lagnado, J. R. (1957). *Experientia* **13**, 476.

Szarkowska, L. and Klingenberg, M. (1963). *Biochem. Z.* **338**, 674.

Tranzer, J. P. and Pearse, A. G. E. (1963). *Nature, Lond.* **199**, 1063.

Von Pechmann, H. and Runge, P. (1894). *Ber. dt. chem. Ges.* **27**, 2920.

Zöllner, N. and Rothermund, E. (1954). *Hoppe-Seyl. Z.* **298**, 97.

DISCUSSION

In reply to a question from DR. RILEY regarding the differing effects of anaerobiosis and cyanide on tetrazolium reduction, DR. SLATER explained that anaerobic conditions prevented the auto-oxidation of reduced ubiquinone, and thus channelled the electron pathway into tetrazolium reduction. In view of the accepted interactions of cyanide with ubiquinones, he agreed that it was difficult to explain the lack of the effect of cyanide on the neo-tetrazolium system, aerobically or anaerobically. DR. HEATH asked Dr. Slater whether he had examined other dehydrogenase systems to ascertain whether the tetrazoliums reacted at the same stages with all systems. DR. SLATER pointed out that this work represented only a small part of his interest, and he had not had an opportunity to extend these studies. However, he had examined the β-hydroxybutyrate-DPN system and in that case reaction occurred mainly at the level of the DPNH-flavoprotein stage.

The Localization of Ubiquinones in the Cornea and Retina

A. G. Everson Pearse

Postgraduate Medical School, London, England

Ubiquinones (UQ) are present in the mitochondria of the corneal stromal cells, and in those of the epithelium and endothelium. In the newborn chick, and throughout early development, they are diffusely distributed in the stroma. A metabolic role in the carriage of electrons through the corneal ground substance is postulated.

In the retina (rat and chick) mitochondrial UQ is present in the various layers much as would be expected from the overall distribution of mitochondria. Additionally, a very much stronger concentration of UQ is present in the outer segments of the rods and cones. Here it is presumed to be dissolved in the lipid of the discs and it is suggested that it may play a role in electron transport along the folded plasma membranes of which the discs are composed.

1. Introduction

The part played in the functioning of the electron transport chain by lipid-soluble, water-insoluble, quinones and quinonoid compounds has been demonstrated conclusively by the work of Slater and his associates and of Green and co-workers (Slater, Colpa-Boonstra and Links, 1961; Green, 1961). Four types of these compounds are known. They are vitamins E, vitamins K_1 and K_2, ubiquinones and plastoquinones. In mammalian tissues the most important are the ubiquinones (UQ), especially UQ_{45} and UQ_{50}. The subscribed numbers refer to the number of carbon atoms in the isoprene side-chains, as shown in the formula below:

Biochemical studies have indicated that most of the UQ in the tissues is localized in the mitochondria, whereas the vitamins E may be intra- or extra-mitochondrial. The levels of these compounds in mammalian tissues have been estimated. The ubiquinones are normally present in much higher concentrations than the vitamins E and the highest levels are in liver, heart muscle and kidney. In tissues such as brain, where very low levels are recorded, it is clear that the cellular distribution and the level per cell is much more important than the absolute level for the whole organ.

Recently a cytochemical method has been developed (Tranzer and Pearse, 1963) which can localize ubiquinones, and some tocopherols, in the tissues. The method was applied to dark and light adapted mammalian and avian eyes, and to the developing eye of the bird, in order to determine the involvement of UQ in the visual process and on the development of the eye.

2. Materials and Methods

The reaction for UQ was carried out as described by Tranzer and Pearse (1963) on eyes taken from White Sussex chicks between 1 and 20 weeks after hatching and from stock albino and hooded rats of average weight 150 g.

Cryostat sections (8 μ) were incubated at 37°C for 30 min and two types of control section were employed. First, sections previously immersed in absolute ethanol at 22°C for 1 hr and, second, normal fresh cryostat sections incubated in the absence of hydroquinone.

Both types of control gave negative results indicating that the substance responsible for the reaction was a redox compound, soluble in ethanol, and not any endogenous protein-bound derivative, such as lipoic acid.

3. Results

Cornea

The results obtained in the cornea of the chick are shown in Plates 1–3. An overall positive reaction (extra-mitochondrial) in the corneal stroma can be observed to fall practically to nothing at the corneo-scleral junction (Plate 1). UQ levels are moderately high in the iris and ciliary muscle and very high in the basal layer of the epithelium. Bowman's membrane is visible on the right and Descemet's membrane is just visible in some places on the left. More information can be obtained from Plates 2 and 3, which cover the whole thickness of the central cornea, leaving out a small intervening layer of stroma. In Plate 2 the high UQ level in the mitochondria of the basal layer of the epithelium is clearly shown. In the individual cells of the stroma the mitochondria are also strongly reactive. In addition, there is a diffuse, non-mitochondrial, reaction in the stromal connective tissues which increases in intensity from without inwards. At the point shown in Plate 2, Bowman's membrane is reactive but towards the periphery (Plate 1) it is not. Descemet's membrane (Plate 3) is apparently everywhere non-reactive. The corneal endothelium shows a fairly strong mitochondrial reaction, as does the lens epithelium below it.

Retina

No significant differences could be detected in the distribution of UQ as between the dark and light-adapted eye but the localization in both chick and rat was interesting in itself. Plate 4 shows UQ in the albino rat eye. Appearances in the chick eye are essentially similar. The ganglion cell and inner plexiform layers show a moderate reaction, individual ganglion cells being quite distinct at high powers of magnification. Low levels are seen in the inner nuclear layer and a rather stronger reaction is present in the outer plexiform layer. The rod and cone nuclei, as expected, react weakly. Most striking is the very high activity in the *outer* rod segments with a much weaker reaction in the inner segments. This is exactly opposite to the localization of the cytochemically demonstrable mitochondrial NADH-diaphorase, and of the coenzyme I linked dehydrogenases. (Cone outer segments, judging by the results in the chick eye, contain much less ubiquinone than those of the rods.)

4. Discussion

Cornea

The dependence of the corneal stroma upon its epithelium, at least with respect to protein synthesis, has been established by the work of Herrmann and Love (1959).

Already Herrmann and Hickman (1948a, b) had shown that lactate, produced in the stroma by glycolysis, could not be further metabolized *in situ*. They considered that oxidation of stromal metabolites was dependent on the functioning epithelium. The sclera, on the other hand, appears to function without any epithelial assistance.

Summing up the results of his own work, and that of others, Herrmann (1961) postulated a transfer of electrons from the stromal cells "through a non-cellular matrix of ground substance of the stromal cells to the epithelial cells". Extending this idea, he developed a tentative scheme involving electron transfer by protein thiol groups in the ground substance to lipoic acid in the epithelium, and thence to the terminal electron transport system.

The results presented above indicate that a diffusely distributed ethanol-soluble redox compound is present in the corneal stroma of the chick eye. Although absolute proof cannot be obtained by cytochemical methods it is probable that this compound belongs to the ubiquinone series. The only reasonable alternative would be one of the tocopherols (vitamins E). In either case the compound could act as an intermediate in the transport of electrons. From the topographical localization of the compound it can be postulated that the flow of electrons could be either from the stromal cells to the epithelium or vice versa, but not to or from the endothelium. This is isolated by the UQ-free membrane of Descemet.

As observed by Herrmann, "the cornea may represent a model system of wider significance for the study of developmental processes". At the present time the cornea is the only mammalian tissue in which diffuse *extracellular* UQ has been observed. In several others, notably the exocrine pancreas and salivary glands, a diffuse intra-cellular reaction accompanies the usual strong mitochondrial reaction.

The transport of electrons from one mitochondrion to another is a process which may take place by a number of different mechanisms, and there is no biochemical evidence to suggest that UQ is concerned. Transmission of electrons through the non-diffusable structural elements of the ground substance of the corneal stroma has been considered essential for the maintenance of amino-acid turnover. It is at least possible that UQ provides this mechanism in the case of the chick cornea.

Retina

The ultrastructure of the rod and cone outer segments has been well described by Sjöstrand (1961), and by De Robertis and Lasansky (1961), Moody and Robertson (1960) and others. In both cases this consists of a series of discs formed by folding of the external plasma membrane. The discs have a characteristic 5-layered structure, the middle layer being composed of two polar lipid molecules with their non-polar ends apposed horizontally.

The cytochemical observations of the present study indicate a high concentration of UQ in the disc region of the rods and cones and, from the known characteristics of UQ it is possible to localize the compound in the lipid zone of the discs. According to Sjöstrand (1961), 40% of the dry weight of the outer segments is lipid.

In the case of the visual cell outer segments, as with the cornea, it is not unreason-able to suggest a metabolic function for UQ in facilitating electron transport through the length of the outer segment and, presumably, thence to the large mitochondria of the inner segment.

If some force exists which maintains the system in the reduced or partially reduced state, then the collection of ubiquinol-loaded discs in the outer segment may act as a charged condenser, discharging on receipt of the appropriate signal.

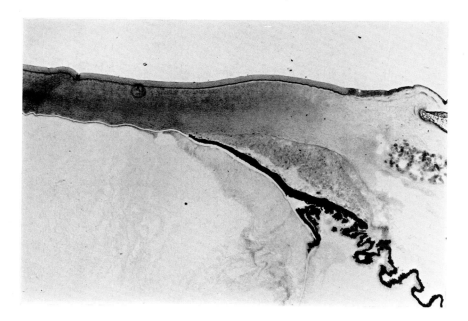

PLATES 1–4. All illustrations are of 8μ fresh frozen (cryostat) sections. Incubated to show the localization of ubiquinone.

PLATE 1. 10-day old chick. Shows (*left*) cornea and (*right*) corneo-scleral junction. A strong diffuse reaction in the former falls to nothing as the sclera is approached. ($\times$ 38)

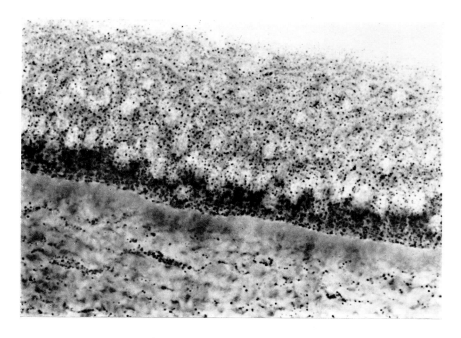

PLATE 2. The corneal epithelium and Bowman's membrane with underlying stroma. Diffusely distributed UQ extends through the membrane. ($\times$ 960)

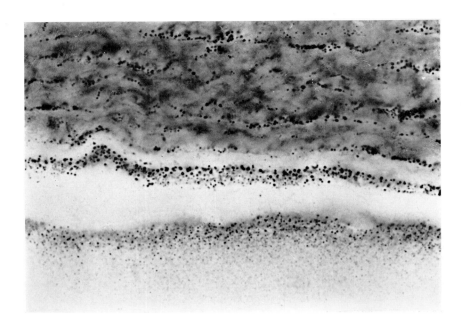

PLATE 3. Below, the lens; above (*middle*) the corneal endothelium, Descemet's membrane, and the stroma. Note the intense diffuse UQ reaction in the latter and its absence from Descemet's membrane. (× 960)

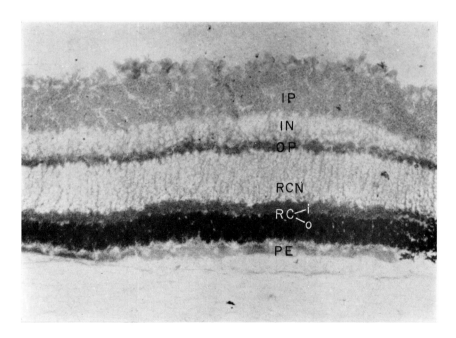

PLATE 4. Albino rat retina. From below upwards, pigment epithelium (PE), outer and inner rod and cone layer (RC), rod and cone nuclei (RCN), outer plexiform (OP), and ganglion cell layers. Note highest activity in the rod and cone outer segments. (× 220)

Abbreviations used: IP, inner plexiform; IN, inner nuclear; OP, outer plexiform; RCN, rod and cone nuclei; RC, rod and cone (inner and outer); PE, pigment epithelium.

Both NADH- and NADPH-diaphorases are present in high concentrations in the outer segment, so that the reduction of ubiquinone by either of the reduced co-enzymes would be possible.

The cytochemical findings of this study require confirmation and amplification. The first procedure must be carried out at the biochemical level with precise identification of the responsible quinone. Microdissection and microassay techniques should confirm the localization indicated by conventional cytochemistry. Beyond this, for both cornea and retina, lies a region accessible to further experiment. Amplification of the role of UQ in corneal and retinal metabolism can confidently be expected.

ACKNOWLEDGMENTS

I have received admirable technical assistance from Mr. J. D. Bancroft, and from Mr. W. Brackenbury who took the photomicrographs.

REFERENCES

De Robertis, E. and Lasansky, A. (1961). In *The Structure of the Eye*, ed. by G. K. Smelser, pp. 29–49. Academic Press, New York.

Green, D. E. (1961). *Quinones and Electron Transport*, pp. 130–160. Ciba Foundation Symposium. Churchill, London.

Herrmann, H. (1961). In *The Structure of the Eye*, ed. by G. K. Smelser, pp. 421–433. Academic Press, New York.

Herrmann, H. and Hickman, F. H. (1948a). *Bull. Johns Hopkins Hosp.* **82**, 255.

Herrmann, H. and Hickman, F. H. (1948b). *Bull. Johns Hopkins Hosp.* **82**, 260.

Herrmann, H. and Love, D. S. (1959). *J. biophys. biochem. Cytol.* **6**, 135.

Moody, M. F. and Robertson, J. D. (1960). *J. biophys. biochem. Cytol.* **7**, 87.

Sjöstrand, F. S. (1961). In *The Structure of the Eye*, ed. by G. K. Smelser, pp. 1–28. Academic Press, New York.

Slater, E. C., Colpa-Boonstra, J. P. and Links, J. (1961). *Quinones in Electron Transport*, pp. 161–189. Ciba Foundation Symposium. Churchill, London.

Tranzer, J. P. and Pearse, A. G. E. (1963). *Nature, Lond.* **199**, 1063.

DISCUSSION

PROFESSOR PEARSE in reply to a question from DR. NEWHOUSE agreed that Dr. Enoch had found no autoreduction of tetrazolium salts in the dark adapted retina, although there was evidence for specific reduction on exposure to light. He felt that this might well support his own proposition of a reduced system poised for release by the light impulse.

DR. MANUEL said he was interested in Professor Pearse's findings in view of the close relationship between the visual cell and photosynthetic sensitivity. He understood that ubiquinones were involved in this latter process and wondered whether Professor Pearse had any information regarding this point. PROFESSOR PEARSE thought that the material to which he was referring was most likely to be plastoquinone, contained in the chloroplasts. He intended to obtain the spadix of the wild arum in the spring, as this was reputed to be rich in ubiquinone.*

PROFESSOR COHEN expressed delight at Professor Pearse's findings and suggested that ubiquinone could well be incorporated into the scheme which he and Professor Noell had indicated on the previous day. In that case the ultimate electron acceptor would be a quinone rather than oxygen. This quinone would provide the 'sink' into which electrons would flow on

*Footnote added in proof: Spring, 1965. Cytochemical confirmation of very high ubiquinone content in *Arum maculatum* spadix.

illumination. With a scheme such as this, he added, one would be able to overcome the problem of the survival of the ERG in anoxia. It seemed plausible that the electrons might be transferred subsequently to oxygen by a slower reaction. PROFESSOR PEARSE agreed that this concept was very exciting, and that it provided a further line of approach to the system he was studying.

In reply to a question from DR. CAMPBELL, PROFESSOR PEARSE referred to work by Folkers suggesting that both vitamins K and E (quasi-substances) might substitute for ubiquinone (veristic-substance) under certain circumstances. He felt, therefore, that although vitamin E did not normally participate in the outer limb system, it might nevertheless exert some protective action when ubiquinones were deficient.

PROFESSOR NOELL reminded the meeting that both ubiquinone and vitamin E were antioxidants, having importance in the indication of muscular dystrophy. He thought that they might well be involved in the mechanism of oxygen poisoning.

DR. AMES suggested that it might be of interest to add hydroquinone to an *in vitro* system and to determine whether this had any effect on the ERG.

DR. CAMPBELL recalled that many years ago she had studied the toxic effects of naphthalene and had observed that this substance was broken down to hydroquinone in the body. Retinal effects appeared some few hours after administration to rabbits. PROFESSOR PEARSE commented on the possibility that the high lipid solubility of naphthalene would contribute to its concentration in the retina.

In closing the discussion on this most interesting paper, DR. FUTTERMAN asked Professor Pearse whether he was convinced personally that this substance was ubiquinone. PROFESSOR PEARSE agreed that his view was based on histochemical evidence, but added that he had made every effort to exclude the possibility of obvious interference by similar substances. Although he was quite sure this would prove to be ubiquinone, he intended to examine the substance in other ways and hoped that other biochemists would attempt to isolate it and characterise it.

A Preliminary Report on the Effects of Hyperoxia on the Alkaline Phosphatases of the Retina

HEATHER A. BROWN, CLIVE N. GRAYMORE AND MARY J. TOWLSON

Department of Pathology, Institute of Ophthalmology, University of London, England

The suggestion that high alkaline phosphatase activity may be associated with the development of the retinal vasculature prompted the present investigation. This enzyme complex has been studied in the kitten and ratling, both during oxygen-induced vaso-obliteration, and also in the subsequent vaso-proliferation which results from returning the animal to air. A number of animals have been subjected to varying periods of hyperoxia, and the alkaline phosphatase activities of their retinas examined, both with regard to total content, and also distribution. The results suggest that 3 days' exposure to atmospheres of 80 – 90% oxygen induces a considerable fall in alkaline phosphatase activity, and that after as little as 6 hr hyperoxia a slight reduction is apparent. The possible association of all, or part, of the enzyme complex with vessel growth is emphasized by the finding that the total alkaline phosphatase content of the retina of the mature cat is only a small fraction of that of the kitten.

Histochemical treatment of flat preparations of rat retina has revealed the presence of high concentrations of alkaline phosphatase in the walls of the arteries and capillary network; these are particularly apparent at the branch points. This distribution confirms the findings of other workers, and supports the hypothesis that the enzyme may play some part in controlling the size of the arterial lumen, possibly by providing a regulatory "sampling" mechanism. The effect of hyperoxia, in depressing the activity of alkaline phosphatase, has been demonstrated histochemically in both ratling and kitten retinas. Quantitative techniques suggest that in the kitten this reduction in total activity is maintained during the vasoproliferative phase which characterises the return of the oxygen-treated animal to air, although intense alkaline phosphatase activity can be shown histochemically in the vasoproliferating regions. The significance of these findings is discussed.

1. Introduction

That hyperoxia induces pathological changes in the vasculature of immature retinas is now well established (see Ashton, 1957a,b). The characteristic vaso-obliterative effect of hyperoxia, and the vasoproliferative phase which ensues on the return of the experimental animal to air, can be demonstrated in the immature retinas of kittens up to 3 weeks of age (Ashton, Ward and Serpell, 1953, 1954; Ashton and Cook, 1954). The implications of these changes, with reference to the human condition, are discussed by Ashton (1954b).

It must be emphasized that the vaso-obliterative effect of hyperoxia is dependent on the stage of immaturity of the retinal tissue, not of the growing vessels *per se.* (Ashton, Ward and Serpell, 1953, 1954 but see Ashton and Pedler, 1962). The precise nature of the change which nullifies the toxic effects of oxygen at maturity, is not yet clearly understood. So far, few investigations of the oxygen-treated retina have revealed any significant biochemical response which might account for the effects of hyperoxia. Hellström (1956) found no change in the activity of succinic dehydrogenase in the retina of oxygen-exposed animals, and no change in the rates of respiration or anaerobic glycolysis of retinas from ratlings maintained from birth in an atmosphere of 70% oxygen. Similarly, Graymore (unpublished observation) found no change in glycolytic or respiratory rates of retinas from kittens subjected to 3 days' hyperoxia,

115

and no change in their rates of glucose uptake or lactic acid production. Furthermore, he found no difference in lactic acid content of retinas from oxygen-treated and control kittens, even when the freshly-dissected retinas were rapidly frozen to minimize any post-mortem changes.* Graymore and Towlson (unpublished observations), measured pyridine nucleotide levels in the retinas of oxygen-treated and control kittens, and found marked changes in the redox potentials of both the di- and tri-phosphopyridine nucleotide systems. The ratio of oxidized to reduced di-phosphopyridine nucleotide changed from 7·7 in untreated animals to 16·9 in animals maintained in oxygen for 3 days. Changes in the tri-phosphopyridine nucleotide system were reversed, the ratio of reduced to oxidized pyridine nucleotide increasing from 3·7 to 7·2. This is interesting in view of the recent report by Chance, Jamieson and Coles (1965), that hyperbaric oxygen can affect the intracellular oxidation-reduction states of reduced pyridine nucleotides in general, and the energy-linked pathway for pyridine nucleotide reduction in particular. Graymore and Towlson (unpublished observation) have also shown an increase in the level of Na/K ATP-ase in hyperoxic animals.

Kojima, Iida and Okada (1960) have reported that the repeated subcutaneous administration of small doses of insulin induces a lowering of the alkaline phosphatase activity of rabbit retinas. Campbell (1937), and Bean, Johnson, Smith and Bauer (1953), have shown that insulin can enhance the general toxic effects of oxygen. Furthermore, Graymore (unpublished observation) found that an intravenous injection of insulin causes immediate and complete closure of all the retinal vessels of a kitten which is already exhibiting partial retinal vaso-obliteration as a result of oxygen treatment. Nilausen (1958) has demonstrated histochemically the intense alkaline phosphatase activity of human foetal retinas, particularly at the periphery of the growing vasculature, and has emphasized its absence from the non-vascularized areas. An investigation of the alkaline phosphatase content of retinas of oxygen-treated and control animals was therefore considered to be of value.

2. Methods

Animals

All animals used in this investigation were reared at the Institute of Ophthalmology. Weaned kittens were maintained on a diet of milk and meat or fish, and rats on the standard diet used routinely by this laboratory (Diet 41, Bruce and Parkes, 1946). Kittens subjected to hyperoxia were less than 12 days old at the beginning of the experiment; the age of survival animals is shown in Table 5. Adult cats were over 6 months old. Ratlings were aged 5–9 days at the start of the experiments and adult rats were aged 3–4 months, unless otherwise stated in the text.

Controls

Wherever possible litter mates were used for control purposes, although in the case of ratling 3-day-experiments, control animals were of a different litter born on the same day. This was necessitated by the fact that it was not found possible in the case of rats to transfer the mother every 12 hr from her "oxygen" litter to her "air" litter without inducing a stress that created a positive hazard.

Oxygenation

The specially constructed incubation chambers for exposure at atmospheric pressure have been described elsewhere (Ashton et al., 1954). The high pressure chamber used in certain experiments was kindly donated by Vickers Research Ltd.

---

* Graymore (1964) did show, however, that the so-called M-isoenzyme of lactic acid dehydrogenase increases markedly in the retina during the proliferative phase.

Preparation of tissue

Adult cats and kittens were killed by the administration of a lethal dose of Nembutal. Adult rats were killed by cervical dislocation, and ratlings by decapitation.

The eyes were removed as rapidly as possible, and the retinas dissected into normal saline. The retinas were homogenized in de-ionized water, using a tissue ratio of 1 retina/ ml of water for kitten retinas, and up to 16 retinas/ml in the case of ratlings.

The homogenates were diluted with an equal volume of water, and aliquots reserved for protein analysis by the microkjeldahl technique. After the addition of 2 drops of chloroform as a preservative, the homogenates were kept for 2 days at 4°C, so that auto-lysis might occur (as recommended by Reis, 1951). Subsequently, the homogenates were centrifuged, and the supernatants used for the estimation of alkaline phosphatase activity.

Quantitative estimation of alkaline phosphatase activity

The method used was that described by Reis (1951) involving the hydrolysis by non-specific alkaline phosphatases, at their optimum pH 9·0, of sodium phenyl phosphate. The inorganic phosphate thus liberated was estimated by the method of Fiske and Subbarow (1925). The optical densities of the resulting blue solutions were read against distilled water in a Hilger Spekker at 680 mμ using filter 8, which previously had been established as the most suitable for the purpose.

Histochemical demonstration of alkaline phosphatase activity

For the histochemical demonstration of alkaline phosphatase activity in the retina, eyes were deep frozen with Cardice, immediately after removal from the animal. They were stored at −20°C until required, when they were allowed to thaw in cold 10% formol saline, and the retinas dissected out. The flat preparations were incubated for 15–20 min in Tris buffer, pH 9·0, containing sodium α-naphthyl phosphate and 5-chloro-ortho-toluidine, (Pearse, 1960) to develop a red-brown colour at the site of alkaline phosphatase activity. They were then drained, mounted and photographed.

A single attempt was also made to inject this reaction mixture into the drained vascular system of a rat, so that the colour could be developed *in situ*.

3. Results

Tables I and II show the effect of 3 days' exposure to 85% oxygen on the total

TABLE I

Effect of 3 days' hyperoxia on alkaline phosphatase activity of kitten retinas

										Mean	S.E.M.	
Control	87·7	85·8	46·1	83·9	172·5	82·6	158·3	180·9	108·0	111·8	± 15·7	(9)
Experimental	73·9	73·0	23·4	80·7	133·1	76·5	82·5	143·0	119·2	89·5	± 12·3	(9)

Results expressed as μg inorganic phosphate released/hr per retina. Number of animals used in parenthesis.

TABLE II

									Mean	S.E.M.
Control	18·0	18·7	9·0	18·3	15·7	17·6	26·3	59·8	22·9	± 5·5
Experimental	15·6	18·5	5·4	19·6	14·8	12·3	13·7	37·4	17·2	± 3·3

As above, but results expressed as μg inorganic phosphate released/hr per mg protein.

alkaline phosphatase activity of kitten retinas. When a ranking technique is employed, to assess the effect of this treatment, it appears that the fall in activity in the treated animals is significant at the 5% level, whether the results are expressed as μg phosphate released/hr/retina, or as μg phosphate/hr/mgm protein.

Table III shows that 3 days' hyperoxia also reduces alkaline phosphatase activity of ratling retinas, although the differences between the mean values are not statistically significant. The results shown in Table IV indicate that, in 2 out of 3 cases examined, ratlings subjected to 6 hr oxygen at 14 lb/in² show a fall in the alkaline phosphatase activity of their retinas.

TABLE III

Effect of 3 days' hyperoxia on alkaline phosphatase activity of ratling retinas

	μg P/hr/mg protein			Mean	S.E.M.	μg P/hr/retina			Mean	S.E.M.
Control	11·3	8·7	16·3	12·1	± 2·2	7·6	6·8	14·0	9·5	± 2·3
Experimental	8·3	5·4	13·9	9·2	± 2·5	6·3	3·7	12·3	7·4	± 2·6

TABLE IV

Effect of 6 hr hyperoxia (14 lb/in²) on alkaline phosphatase activity of ratling retinas

	μg P/hr/mg protein			μg P/hr/retina		
Control	3·6	5·3	7·3	1·5	2·1	5·2
Experimental	3·0	4·4	9·2	1·2	1·4	6·6

TABLE V

Effect of hyperoxia and subsequent survival on alkaline phosphatase activity of kitten retinas

Experiment 1		Experiment 2	
4-day-old control	175·5	8-day-old control	132·0
6 hr oxygen	140·3	5·5 hr oxygen	138·9
18-day-old control	147·8	11-day-old control	180·9
3 days oxygen + 11 days survival	} 100·5	3 days oxygen	143·0
		28-day-old control	175·5
		3 days oxygen + 17 days survival	} 129·0

Results expressed as μg inorganic phosphate released/hr/retina

Table V gives the results of some experiments in which kittens were subjected to 85% oxygen for the periods quoted. Experiment 1 shows that after as little as 6 hr treatment, a fall in alkaline phosphatase activity was detectable, although in experiment 2 there was no observable effect at 5·5 hr. Those kittens subjected to 3 days' hyperoxia followed by a survival period in air, had not regained the control level of activity, even after 17 days.

The retinas of adult rats and cats were found to have much lower alkaline phosphatase activities than did immature retinas from the same species. The enzyme activity (expressed as μg phosphate released/hr per mg protein) of retinas from 10-day-old rats was found to be 12·8, whereas the corresponding figure for adult rats was 2·6. The mean normal value for kitten retinas was 23·0 whereas two adult cats were found to have retinal alkaline phosphatase activities of 0·7 and 1·6. Statistical analysis of results revealed a correlation between enzyme activity of untreated rat retinas and age. There was a significant positive correlation ($r = +0·677$; $P > 0·10$, $< 0·05$) between alkaline phosphatase activity and age up to 12 days: rats aged from 48 to 120 days showed a significant negative correlation ($r = -0·963$; $P > 0·10$, $< 0·05$) between the two. No significant correlation between age and alkaline phosphatase activity of normal kitten retinas could be found, although the drastic fall in activity shown by adult cat retinas has been mentioned already.

Histochemical treatment of flat retinal preparations corroborated in general the quantitative findings; alkaline phosphatase activity in the normal 11-day-old kitten was most intense in the vascular region and the staining appeared to outline the vessels. In the retina of the oxygen treated 11-day-old kitten, alkaline phosphatase activity was greatly reduced and no vessels were visible.

In the retina of the 28-day kitten alkaline phosphatase activity appeared to be distributed more evenly than in the 3-day kitten and the staining was not so markedly restricted to the vascularized region, although the vessel walls still seemed to be the major sites of enzyme activity. The retina of an 8-day kitten, subjected to 3 days hyperoxia and then allowed to survive for 17 days, showed extensive vaso-proliferation and the regions of vaso-proliferation appeared to have a high level of alkaline phosphatase activity, concentrated around the zone of *active* vessel growth. This observation contrasted with the quantitative estimations which showed a reduced overall level of activity at this time.

Histochemical treatment of the retina of a normal 7-day rat revealed intense alkaline phosphatase activity both in the vessel walls and in the immediately surrounding tissue. On the other hand, the retina of a rat of the same age which had received 3 days' hyperoxia prior to investigation showed a considerable reduction in activity in the tissue and a loss both of the smaller capillaries and the associated staining.

Examination of the retina of the intravitally stained retina revealed more intense alkaline phosphatase activity in the branch points and small vessels than in the main vessels. A number of technical difficulties connected with this process have so far prevented any further investigation in this direction.

4. Discussion

It should be stressed that investigations on the kitten retina were severely hampered by lack of material, necessitating studies on smaller groups than would otherwise be demanded. Nevertheless, a decreased level of alkaline phosphatase activity of the immature retina appears to be induced by hyperoxia both in ratlings and kittens, although the present results suggest that it may not be an invariable consequence of this treatment.

Unless the vasculature of one of each pair of retinas is examined by injection technique it is not possible to guarantee that adequate vaso-obliteration has occurred.

Shortage of material prohibited such action in the present series. Variations, both as regards the susceptibility or well-being of the animals, as well as the maintenance of adequate oxygen tensions, are to be expected, and should be taken into account when judging these results. Nevertheless, it seems fairly clear that hyperoxia induces a fall in activity of the alkaline phosphatases of the immature retina of the ratling and of the kitten. It is not yet certain, however, whether this fall is the cause of the observed vascular changes or conversely, whether it results from the disruption of the normal vascular pattern. In this respect, the observation by Ashton and Pedler (1962) that endothelial changes occur as early as 6 hr. after treatment is relevant, and the present results do little to invalidate the possibility that the observed changes could be a result rather than a cause. The connection between endothelial cells and alkaline phosphatases has been stressed repeatedly (Nilausen, 1958; Romanul and Bannister, 1962; Kuwabara and Cogan, 1963). It would be of interest to measure the activity of the retinas of animals which have had less than 6 hr hyperoxia, and in which the endothelial cells have not yet been shown to degenerate.

Nilausen (1958) has emphasized the alkaline phosphatase activity of the cells at the periphery of the growing retinal vessel system. It has been suggested (Ashton, 1954b) that these cells may be mesenchymal precursors of the vessels. The present investigation has demonstrated histochemically how the activity of this tissue is diminished during hyperoxia. In the vasoproliferative retina, the intense activity which is revealed by histochemical techniques is not paralleled by the results of quantitative estimations which suggest that the low levels of alkaline phosphatase activity, induced by hyperoxia, are maintained to some extent in the survival kitten retina. It is possible, of course, that, although the alkaline phosphatase activity demonstrated histochemically is intense, it is also limited and restricted in area, thus contributing little to the total value.

It is also possible that the reduced alkaline phosphatase activity in survival animals, as shown by determinations of total activity, may reflect some permanent injury to the system, this being the cause of the ensuing chaotic and unrestrained vessel re-development.

It cannot be emphasized too strongly that the term "alkaline phosphatase" covers a multiplicity of enzymes which, while sharing a common ability to hydrolyse phosphoric esters, may have widely differing functions and properties *in vivo*. It may be that oxygen affects various components of the alkaline phosphatase complex in different ways. Separation and study of the "isoenzymes" of alkaline phosphatase may help to elucidate which components of this complex are affected by oxygen, and to what extent.

The positive correlation which exists between alkaline phosphatase activity and age in the ratling retina up to at least the 12th day, is interesting in view of the developmental pattern of the retinal vasculature. In the rat, a primitive capillary net is formed initially in the nerve fibre layer, from arteries and veins radiating symmetrically from the central vessels at the optic disc. By the 11th day, the superficial vascular layer is complete, the peripheral vessels maturing last. The deep capillary net, which begins to form at the 8th to 9th day, is complete by the 15th day, at which stage the retina has achieved the adult vascular pattern (Ashton and Blach, 1961). It seems possible that the alkaline phosphatase activity reflects the development of new ramifications of the capillary network. In this respect it would be of interest to examine the alkaline phosphatase activity after the 15th day, when the mature arrangement has been reached. It has been shown that a statistically significant negative correlation exists between alkaline phosphatase activity and age between 48 and 120 days, but estimations of the alkaline phosphatase activity of retinas of rats from 13 to 47 days of age have yet to be attempted.

Although the adult cat retina appears to have an extremely low alkaline phosphatase activity, when compared with that of the immature retina, no significant correlation could be found between activity and age from 5 to 28 days. This inability to correlate the two factors in the kitten, as opposed to the ratling, may be due to the relative variability of the control values in the kitten. A similar problem was encountered by Finegan (1964) who measured the concentration of alkaline phosphatase in the juxtaglomerular apparatus of the rat, and found that the observed activity varied with the strain of the rat used. Although the rats in the present investigation were all of the same strain, the cats of course were not, and this may explain the difficulty in obtaining a standard control figure.

The precise function of the alkaline phosphatase of the retina is, at present, open to speculation. Romanul and Bannister (1962) have assigned a "sampling" role to these enzymes, in view of their concentration at the origin of arteries and arterioles from larger vessels. They also point out the absence of alkaline phosphatases from the venous side of the circulation, and suggest that the size of the lumen of arteries is continually being regulated, in response to the sampling of the chemical content of the blood by the alkaline phosphatases. Samorajski and McCloud (1961) have also observed that an increased transmitting function across the blood-brain barrier can be correlated with an increase in alkaline phosphatase activity in the vascular endothelium.

It is interesting to note that, after retinal detachment, not only does hyperoxia have no further vaso-obliterative effect, but the vessels which are already closed reopen (depending, of course, on the duration of the closure) (Ashton and Cook, 1954). It can be argued that this results from the lower oxygen tensions attendant on the separation of the retina from the choroidal circulation; or, on a purely mechanical basis, it could result from the release of tension inside the retina. To clarify this point, an investigation into the alkaline phosphatase content of the detached retina would be of value.

Why it is that only the growing vessels of the immature retina are affected by hyperoxia is still a matter of conjecture. It has been suggested (Ashton, 1954a; Ashton et al., 1954), that the differences in radial size, vascularization and metabolic rate of the immature and adult tissues may account for their different degrees of susceptibility. In this connection, it is of interest that Hellström and Nergårdh (1963) have successfully used hypothermia to protect new-born mice from the general effects of hyperoxia, and they conclude that the decreased metabolic needs, during hypothermia, protect the retina which is suffering from impaired energy production during exposure to oxygen.

The experiments described in this paper must be considered to comprise merely a preliminary investigation into the complex reactions of alkaline phosphatases, and the effects of hyperoxia on their activity in the immature retina.

ACKNOWLEDGMENTS

The authors wish to express their gratitude to the Royal National Institute for the Blind for financial assistance towards this project. They also thank Professor Norman Ashton for his continued encouragement, and the excellent technical assistance of Mr. Ralph Kissun is gratefully acknowledged.

REFERENCES

Ashton, N. H. (1954a). *Tran. Am. Acad. Ophthal. Oto-lar.* **58**, 51.

Ashton, N. H. (1954b). *Br. J. Ophthal.* **38**, 385.

Ashton, N. H. (1957a). *Ann. Rev. Med.* **8**, 441.

Ashton, N. H. (1957b). *Am. J. Ophthal.* **44**, pt. II, 7.

Ashton, N. H. and Blach, R. (1961). *Br. J. Ophthal.* **45**, 321.

Ashton, N. H. and Cook, C. (1954) *Br. J. Ophthal.* **38**, 433.

Ashton, N. H. and Pedler, C. M. H. (1962). *Br. J. Ophthal.* **46**, 257.

Ashton, N. H., Ward, B. and Serpell, G. (1953). *Br. J. Ophthal.* **37**, 513.

Ashton, N. H., Ward, B. and Serpell, G. (1954). *Br. J. Ophthal.* **38**, 397.

Bean, J. W., Johnson, P., Smith, C. and Bauer, R. (1953). *Fed. Proc.* **12**, 12.

Bruce, H. M. and Parkes, A. S. (1946). *J. Hyg., Camb.* **44**, 501.

Campbell, J. A. (1937). *J. Physiol.* **90**, 91P.

Chance, B., Jamieson, D. and Coles, H. (1965). *Nature, Lond.* **206**, 257.

Finegan, R. P. (1964). *Nature, Lond.* **203**, 768.

Fiske, C. H. and Subbarow, Y. (1925). *J. biol. Chem.* **66**, 357.

Graymore, C. N. (1964). *Nature, Lond.* **201**, 615.

Hellström, B. (1956). *Acta path. microbiol. scand.* **39**, (1) 8.

Hellström, B. and Nergårdh, A. (1963). *Exp. Eye Res.* **2**, 331.

Kojima, K., Iida, M. and Okada, S. (1960). *Acta Soc. ophthal. jap.* **64**, 768.

Kojima, K., Iida, M. and Okada, S. (1961). *Zbl. Ges. Ophthal.* **81**, 181.

Kuwabara, Y. and Cogan, D. G. (1963). *Arch. Ophthal.* **69**, 492.

Nilausen, K. (1958). *Acta Ophthal.* **36**, 65.

Pearse, E. A. G. (1960). *"Histochemistry"* 2nd edit., p. 872., J. and A. Churchill, London.

Reis, J. L. (1951). *Biochem. J.* **48**, 548.

Romanul, F. and Bannister, R. (1962). *Nature, Lond.* **193**, 611.

Samorajski, T. and McCloud, J. (1961). *Lab. Invest.* **10**, 492.

DISCUSSION

The chairman (DR. FUTTERMAN) in opening the discussion expressed pleasure that two different disciplines, those of histochemistry as well as more conventional biochemical techniques, should be applied to a single problem.

DR. KUWABARA added that in his own laboratory he had found that proliferation of the endothelial cells during R.L.F. was associated with an increase in alkaline phosphatase activity. His experiments had shown, also, however, that there was an increase in acid phosphatase, ATP-ase and of glycogen synthesis. It seemed, therefore, that there was a general increase in metabolic activity during this phase. MISS BROWN agreed that it would be reasonable to expect some degree of chemical hyperactivity during such an active phase.

PROFESSOR WALD questioned the advisability of examining such non-specific systems as those of ATP-ase and acid and alkaline phosphatases, as it was very difficult to interpret the real significance of any findings obtained. MISS BROWN pointed out that her results were essentially preliminary and exploratory, and were part of an investigation into a most complex field of which little was known.

In answer to a question from DR. HEATH, MISS BROWN explained that the period of autolysis was required to leach out the enzymes from the sub-cellular particles.

In reply to a comment by DR. TOWLSON on the possible relationship of alkaline phosphatase and glycogen synthesis in mitotic division, PROFESSOR COHEN referred to the finding that a bacterial alkaline phosphatase had been shown to be under repressive control by inorganic phosphate. It could be that this was the linkage, i.e., that both activities indicated a low concentration of inorganic phosphate. It might, therefore, be of value to investigate the level of inorganic phosphate in the tissue during the vaso-proliferative phase.

Metabolic Factors in Diabetic Retinopathy*

HARRY KEEN AND C. CHLOUVERAKIS

Department of Medicine, Guy's Hospital, London, England

The effects of the metabolic disturbance of diabetes mellitus in man have been studied in a variety of tissues. Retina has certain distinctive metabolic properties which might seem to make it specially vulnerable in the disease and it is tempting to attribute the morphological changes so characteristic of long-standing diabetes to such a biochemical mechanism. Experimental studies along these lines, which will be reviewed, have cast little light upon a possible biochemical basis for diabetic retinopathy.

Observations relating to glucose uptake by isolated retina from normal and diabetic animals will be presented with consideration of the role of various chemical and hormonal factors. An inhibitory influence of plasma from severe human diabetics upon normal retina has been demonstrated and will be discussed in relation to similar activity in plasma from patients with renal failure. We have explored the possibility, arising from the work of Randle and his colleagues, that a block of glucose dissimilation in the diabetic is produced by the high circulating levels of non-esterified fatty acids (NEFA) in the disease. Studies of NEFA metabolism in normal and diabetic retina showed that the mechanism described by Randle did not appear to operate but new information on lipid metabolism was obtained and will be described. Studies with ^{14}C-labelled palmitic acid-albumin complex showed a high turnover of fatty acid in the tissue, and the metabolic fat of the radioactive carbon has been followed. In the normal, only about 5% of ingoing NEFA was oxidized to CO_2, but diabetic retina showed a markedly enhanced rate of $^{14}CO_2$ production.

The possibility that this enhanced oxidation of NEFA represents an adaptive change in the tissue of the diabetic animal is being explored. While the adaptation may be to the high circulating fatty acid levels characteristic of diabetes, it is possible that increased glucose dissimilation, stimulated by prolonged hyperglycaemia, may lead to the same end effect. Observations upon such an adaptation to chronic hyperglycaemia and its possible morphological consequences will be discussed.

Despite great advances in knowledge of carbohydrate metabolism and the action of insulin and other hormones, we are little further forward in our understanding of the origins of the clinical syndrome of diabetes mellitus in man. We are departing from the view that it is simply a consequence of insulin lack and the situation is at present one of great complexity. If our knowledge of the causes of diabetes is limited, our understanding of the consequences of the disease is hardly more satisfactory.

Disorders of the eyes, the kidneys, the nerves and the blood vessels appear to be almost inescapable consequences of long-term diabetes in man (Aarseth, 1953; Lundbaek, 1953). Of these, diabetic retinopathy is a major source of disability and ranks high among the causes of blindness.

All varieties of spontaneous diabetes mellitus in man and some forms of secondary diabetes provide conditions favouring the eventual appearance of retinopathy (Bastenie, Pirart and Franckson, 1959; Duncan, MacFarlane and Robson, 1958; *Lancet*, 1959). Little, other than passage of time, seems to be necessary for its development although circumstantial evidence suggests that the rate is faster in the poorly controlled diabetic, that is to say in the person exposed for longer times to higher blood sugar levels. Evaluation of the effect of diabetic control on the march of

* This work was supported by grant A–6135 Met of the U.S. Public Health Service.

retinopathy is difficult for, clearly, a controlled experimental approach involving the deliberate withholding of optimal treatment from patients with established diabetes is not possible. Comparisons which have been made of better and worse controlled patients within a treated group have usually shown the latter at a disadvantage (Dunlop, 1954; Engleson, 1954; Hardin, Jackson, Johnston and Kelly, 1956; Johnsson, 1960). However, this higher incidence may be related less to poor control itself than to some inherent property of the diabetes which gives rise to it. In any case, the relationship has not been observed consistently (Brown and Jones, 1964; Scott, 1953). Therapeutic measures directed to the treatment of retinopathy itself have been offered in abundance but they have added little to our knowledge of the pathogenic mechanisms involved. A striking clinical observation recently published by Powell and Field (1964), however, deserves some attention in this respect. These authors showed that the incidence of retinopathy was much below expectation in diabetics with rheumatoid arthritis who had probably been treated over long periods with salicylates. The significance of their finding is heightened by the comments of Mooney (1963) and others (Esmann, Jensen and Lundbaek, 1963) who have reported regression of retinopathy in diabetics treated with para-aminosalicylic acid preparations. The brief vogues and enthusiasms for a wide variety of treatments in the past emphasises that one must exercise caution in assessing the response of diabetic retinopathy to therapy. In a trial to test therapeutic claims which had been made for vitamin B12 (Keen and Smith, 1959) there was striking evidence of the labile nature of the various elements of the retinopathy. Over the course of a year's close observation, the disappearance of established lesions and the appearance of new lesions was recorded. Similar conclusions regarding the ebb and flow of the retinopathy have been reached by others using different approaches (Becker, Maengwyn-Davies, Rosen, Friedenwald and Winter, 1954; Caird and Garratt, 1962; Lawrence, 1949).

Investigative approaches to diabetic retinopathy have, so far, been mainly along morphological lines, but although there is now broad agreement on the nature of the structural disturbance, there is a wide variety of surmises as to how they arise (Ashton, 1958, 1959; Ballantyne and Loewenstein, 1944; Bloodworth, 1962; Blumenthal, Alex and Goldenberg, 1961; Cogan, Toussaint and Kuwabara, 1961; Cogan and Kuwabara, 1963; Coleman, Becker, Canaan and Rosenbaum, 1962; Pope, 1960). Basically, these fall into two major groups; those which view the retinopathy as the ocular expression of a generalized small vessel disease in diabetes and those which see the vascular disease of the eye as a sequel to special metabolic conditions arising in the diabetic retina. It is with the latter possibility that we have chiefly concerned ourselves.

A deterrent to the experimental study of the pathogenic mechanisms is the long 'incubation period' of diabetic retinopathy—the 5–10 years of diabetes which elapse before clinically recognizable changes occur in the retina. This suggests the operation of subtle, small influences over a long period of time rather than large deviations from the normal which may be readily amenable to laboratory investigation. Another obstacle is the failure, despite the sporadic claims of its occurrence (Hausler, Sibay and Campbell, 1964; Levene, Robertson, Foglia and Singer, 1963; Musacchio, Palermo and Rodriguez, 1964), to produce a morphologically acceptable model retinopathy in animals; a dissimilarity in tissue response to diabetes which counsels even more than the usual caution in carrying over findings in animals to the disease in man.

Although the metabolism of retina has received much attention, few studies have been specially related to the effects of diabetes. With this in mind, studies of glucose

uptake of isolated dog retina were made at the National Institute of Health, U.S.A.*
Eyes were removed immediately after death following exsanguination under light Nembutal anaesthesia and stored on ice. Portions of retina weighing about 40 mg were incubated at 38°C for 90 min in Krebs-Ringer bicarbonate buffer (Umbreit, Burris and Stauffer, 1964) or blood plasma under an atmosphere of 95% O_2 5% CO_2. Glucose and other substances were added as required. The rate of glucose uptake, estimated from its disappearance from the medium during incubation, was found to be approximately linear over an incubation period of 4·5 hr. It was little affected

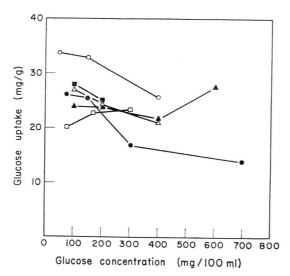

FIG. 1. Glucose uptake by normal dog retina '*in vitro*' incubated in Krebs-Ringer bicarbonate buffer containing glucose at concentrations shown in abscissa. Each point is the mean uptake of three pieces of retina from the same animal, incubated for 90 min.

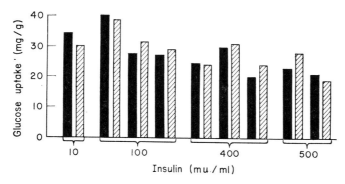

FIG. 2. Influence of insulin (*oblique-shaded columns*) on glucose uptake at various concentrations of hormone. Each column represents the mean of triplicate estimates and each pair of columns is derived from retinal tissue from a single animal.

by up to 3 hrs' storage on ice before incubation started. Raising the glucose concentration of the medium much above 250 mg% had little effect on the rate of glucose uptake by the tissue and in some experiments there was a fall in uptake at the highest concentrations (Fig. 1). When retina was incubated in the presence of growth

* Results reported to 1961 Annual Conference of the American Diabetes Association, New York.

hormone (0·5 mg/ml), epinephrine (0·1 mg/ml), urea (2·5 mg/ml) or cortisol (0·1 mg/ml), only the last showed a small but statistically significant stimulation of glucose uptake.

Crystalline bovine insulin, added to the incubation medium at a variety of concentrations failed to influence glucose uptake of normal dog retina (Fig. 2). Sensitivity to insulin was not shown by retinas of 2 dogs hypophysectomized 10 days before, nor did their rate of glucose uptake differ from normals (Fig. 3).

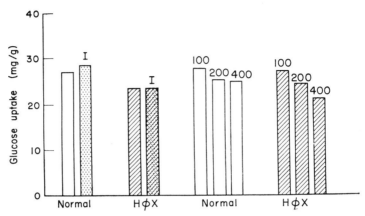

FIG. 3. Influence of insulin (*stippled columns headed I*) and medium glucose concentration (*concentration in mg/100 ml shown above columns*) in normal (*unshaded*) and hypophysectomized (*oblique-shaded*) dog retina (*means of triplicate estimates*).

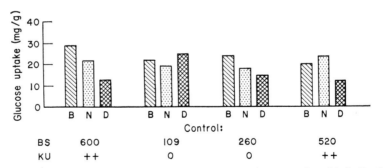

FIG. 4. Glucose uptake by normal dog retina (estimated in triplicate) incubated in buffer (B), normal human plasma (N) and diabetic plasma (D). Preparation of plasma described in text. BS indicates the blood sugar of the diabetic patient at the time plasma was taken and KU the degree of ketonuria. Uptakes from N and D plasma only differ significantly ($P < 0.05$) in first and last sets of columns.

Figure 4 depicts the effect of incubating normal dog retina in heparinized plasma from an uncontrolled diabetic patient compared with a normal, non-diabetic control. Both plasmas were brought to glucose concentrations of about 250 mg/100 ml by 1/2 dilution with buffer and the addition, where necessary, of glucose. Glucose uptake of retina in plasma taken from the diabetic during a period of bad control was markedly less than that in the normal plasma or in buffer. As the patient's control was improved, so this uptake inhibiting effect disappeared but it once again returned as control was lost. This patient also suffered from renal disease due to his diabetes.

With each deterioration in diabetic control there was worsening of the renal failure with elevation of the blood urea. When retina was incubated in the plasma from a non-diabetic patient with terminal renal failure due to glomerulonephritis, similar inhibitory properties were found. However, after the two inhibitory plasmas were dialysed for 24 hr against Krebs-Ringer bicarbonate buffer, the inhibitory effect of the non-diabetic renal failure plasma lessened considerably while that of the diabetic plasma hardly changed (Table I). The presence of this inhibitory activity was found in a number of plasmas from ketotic diabetic patients but was absent from others (Table II).

TABLE I

Inhibitory effect of plasma from patients with diabetic and renal acidosis, on glucose uptake by normal dog retina before and after dialysis
(% of uptake of accompanying normal)

	Before dialysis (%)	After dialysis (%)
Diabetic	63·2	54·0
Renal	48·4	86·7

TABLE II

Direct comparison of glucose uptake by normal dog retina incubated in plasma from normal and uncontrolled diabetic patients (mg/g retina/90 min)
(medium concentration adjusted as described in text)

Normal	Diabetic	D/N(%)
21·8 ± 4·3	13·3 ± 0·6	61
28·1 ± 4·7	20·8 ± 2·5	74
28·1 ± 4·7	30·3 ± 2·8	107
17·3 ± 0·5	21·8 ± 1·9	126
17·3 ± 0·5	14·4 ± 1·1	83
28·5 ± 1·2	20·4 ± 1·4	72
28·5 ± 1·2	22·4 ± 0·5	77

These experiments confirmed the insensitivity of glucose uptake of retina to insulin. They suggested that very high concentrations of glucose *per se* or the presence of some circulating inhibitory factor in diabetic plasma might restrict glucose uptake by retina and so perhaps initiate changes in this highly glucose dependent tissue (Ames and Gurian, 1963).

At this time, the formulation of Randle's hypothesis of the glucose-fatty acid cycle suggested a possible explanation of the inhibitory effect of diabetic plasma. Randle and his colleagues demonstrated, in certain tissues, that raised concentrations of non-esterified fatty acid (NEFA) and ketone bodies impeded glucose breakdown (Randle, Garland, Hales and Newsholme, 1963). It seemed possible that plasma from the poorly controlled diabetic owed its inhibitory activity to its high levels of circulating NEFA or NEFA metabolites (Schrade, Boehle, Biegler and Harmuth, 1963, Werk and Knowles, 1961). Thus, we (Chlouverakis and Keen, 1964; Keen and Chlouverakis, 1964) turned our attention to studies of retinal NEFA metabolism.

Methods

The retinas used were isolated from male Wistar albino rats weighing between 140 and 200 g. Retinas were removed in chilled buffer from the excised globes of animals killed by decapitation after overnight fasting. In general, 1–4 retinas were used in each incubation unit (Keen, Field and Pastan, 1963) each experimental variable being represented by at least three such incubation units. Usually, 0·25 ml of medium was allotted per retina though volumes were adjusted for longer incubations. A series of complexes of crystalline bovine albumin with varying quantities of palmitic acid containing a constant trace of radioactive palmitate labelled with ^{14}C in the C-1 position was prepared. Thus a constant albumin concentration of 3 g/100 ml in the medium could be maintained while varying NEFA concentrations from below 0·2 to over 2 mequiv./l. The suspending fluid was Krebs-Ringer bicarbonate buffer and to this, other substances such as the NEFA albumin complex, glucose and insulin were added as required. All incubations were carried out in a gently shaking incubator at 38°C. Uptakes were calculated from the difference in medium concentration between tissue-containing and tissue-free flasks. CO_2 was collected into a phenylethylamine solution (Woeller, 1961) injected into the centre well or vial base of the incubation unit at the completion of the experiment. Lipids were extracted from medium by the method of Dole (1956) or Dole and Meinertz (1960) and from tissue by homogenizing either in Dole's extraction mixture or in the chloroform methanol solvent of Folch, Lees and Stanley, (1957). Tissue NEFA was separated from fat esters with alkaline ethanol by a modification (Kerpel, Shafrir and Shapiro, 1961) of the method of Borgström (1952). All radioactive samples were counted in a liquid scintillation counter with a diphenyloxazole/dioxane mixture as phosphor.

Results and Discussion

In the absence of information on the metabolism of NEFA by isolated retina, our initial experiments were framed to define the basic behaviour of the normal tissue, and to answer the question 'does isolated retina utilize fatty acid?'. During a 90-min incubation with NEFA-albumin complex and glucose, in all cases labelled palmitate disappeared from the incubation medium (Fig. 5). However, total NEFA in the

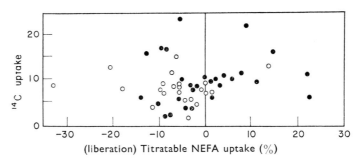

FIG. 5. NEFA 'uptake' from incubation medium expressed as % of initial content; comparison of uptake measured by change in [^{14}C]palmitate in medium (*ordinate*) and by change in Dole extractable titratable acidity (*abscissa*). Washed extracts were treated before titration and counting with an equal volume of distilled water. (○) Unwashed extract; (●) washed extract.

same Dole extracts of medium determined by titration indicated an apparent liberation of NEFA into the incubation medium. This paradoxical effect was probably due to the extraction along with NEFA of a small proportion of the lactate produced by the retina. A single wash of the Dole extracts reduced the apparent NEFA concentration of tissue-containing media, and using the procedure of Dole and Meinertz in which the heptane phase was washed free of lactic acid with blank lower phase there was a clearly demonstrable progressive uptake with time of both radioactivity and of titratable acidity (Fig. 6). However, the early uptake of radioactivity exceeded that of titratable acidity and suggested an initial rapid exchange between tissue and medium NEFA.

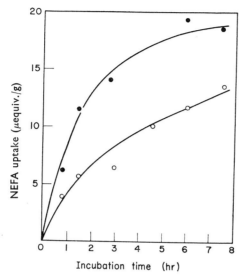

Fig. 6. Time course of NEFA uptake from incubation medium (μequiv./g tissue) estimated on basis of change in medium titratable acidity of lactate-free extracts (○—○) and the disappearance of ^{14}C radioacivity × 1/s.a. from the extracts (●—●).

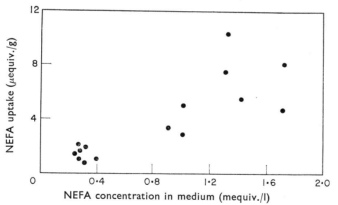

Fig. 7. Relationship between concentration of NEFA in medium (*abscissa*) and rate of uptake by retina (*ordinate*). Uptake in μequiv./g calculated from disappearance of radioactivity from the medium and the specific radioactivity of the preparation.

The fact that this disappearance of NEFA represented a specific uptake of palmitate rather than permeation of the intact albumin-palmitate complex into the tissue was shown by incubating retina in medium in which [^{125}I]albumin was substituted for [^{14}C]NEFA labelled albumin. Under the usual incubation conditions only a very small proportion of the [^{125}I]albumin was to be found in the rinsed tissue—less than one-tenth of the demonstrated palmitate disappearance.

The rate of influx of NEFA into the tissue, calculated from the disappearance of

I

radioactivity from the medium and the specific radioactivity of the NEFA complex used (radioactivity/unit weight of titratable NEFA) is shown in Fig. 7 to rise progressively with increasing medium NEFA concentration over a range resembling that met in human plasma.

The fate of the ingoing labelled palmitate was followed by extraction of the retina in Dole's mixture at the end of incubation. A proportion of the ingoing radioactivity (about 10%) entered the free fatty acid pool of the tissue (Fig. 8), leading to an initial

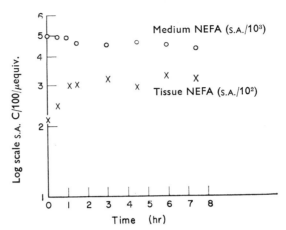

FIG. 8. Changes in the specific radioactivity of NEFA in medium and tissue over a 7·5 hr incubation. There is a tenfold difference in tissue and medium values as plotted (as indicated by the figures in parentheses).

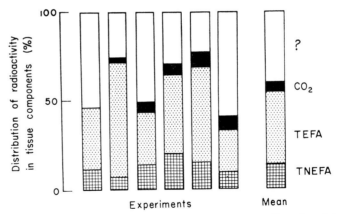

FIG. 9. % representation of radioactivity disappearing from the medium found in tissue NEFA (TNEFA), tissue esterified fat (TEFA) and carbon dioxide (CO_2) following extraction of incubated retina by Dole's method. The portion labelled ? indicates the proportion of ingoing radioactivity unaccounted for 6 individual experiments and their mean is shown.

rapid rise of specific radioactivity. This rise was accounted for entirely by the entrance of the radioactive label into the pool for the total tissue NEFA, determined by titration, did not change significantly throughout the experiment. The succeeding slower rise in tissue NEFA specific radioactivity did not approach that of the incubation medium even after a 7-hr-incubation period.

The fractional distribution of radioactivity in the tissue components examined in several experiments is summarized in Fig. 9. The largest part, 40%, was incorporated into tissue fat ester, about 10–15% of the influx was found in the tissue NEFA pool; and between 5 and 10% was oxidized to CO_2. Thus, about 40% of the ingoing labelled palmitate was unaccounted for.

However, when the tissue was extracted by the Folch procedure into chloroform-methanol the whole measured influx could be recovered. ^{14}C-labelled polar lipids had been discarded in the aqueous phase of the Dole extraction and they were shown by thin layer chromatography to be principally phospholipids (Plate 1). Incorporation into phospholipid claimed a much higher proportion of the ingoing NEFA at lower influx rates than at higher (Fig. 10).

Glucose concentration in the incubation medium markedly influenced NEFA influx. Figure 11 shows that as glucose concentration rose so did the influx of labelled palmitate and the incorporation of radioactivity into tissue lipid.

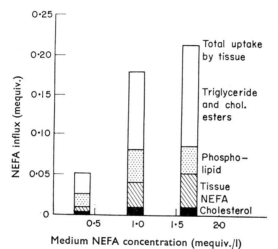

FIG. 10. Distribution of ingoing [14C]palmitate into tissue lipid fractions as indicated, separated by thin layer chromatography.

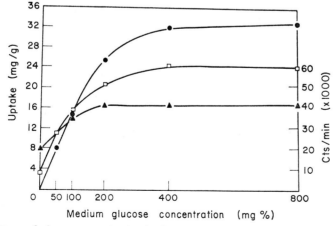

FIG. 11. Influence of glucose concentration in the incubation medium upon rates of glucose uptake (-●-●-); [14C]palmitate uptake (-□-□-); and 14C incorporation into Folch extractable tissue lipid (-▲-▲-). Each estimate represents the mean of three replicates.

Table III shows that glucose uptake rates did not vary over the range of NEFA concentrations examined, suggesting that the mechanism described by Randle and colleagues did not operate in isolated rat retina. No significant effect of insulin upon NEFA influx or glucose uptake was found (Fig. 12).

TABLE III

Influence of medium NEFA concentration on glucose uptake by normal rat retina

NEFA concentration (μequiv./ml)	Glucose uptake (mg/g per 90 min)	No. of experiments
0·2 — 0·4	31·73 ± 1·76	17
0·7 — 0·9	29·73 ± 3·66	7
1·3 — 1·8	31·57 ± 2·26	13

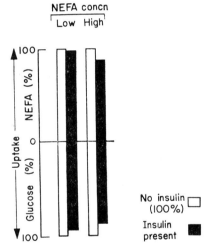

FIG. 12. Effect of insulin (0·1 unit/ml) on NEFA uptake (at low and high medium NEFA concentrations) and upon glucose uptake (at low and high medium NEFA concentrations). In each case, uptake in the absence of insulin (□) is expressed as 100%.

Table IV compares these various aspects of NEFA metabolism in normal retina with retina from alloxan diabetic rats. The duration of diabetes in these animals was comparatively short, varying from 1 to 4 weeks, and there was also considerable

TABLE IV

Comparison of behaviour of retina from normal and diabetic rats

Variable compared	Diabetic as % of normal	No. of experiments	Significance of difference
Glucose uptake	98·8	18	n.s.
Lactate production	99·7	9	n.s.
NEFA influx	113·2	24	n.s.
^{14}C in tissue fat	99·7	27	n.s.
^{14}C in tissue NEFA	96·3	24	n.s.
$^{14}CO_2$ production	173·1	34	$P = 0.02$

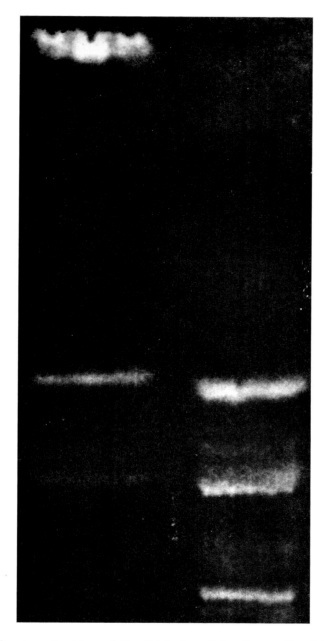

PLATE 1. Radioautograph picture of the distribution of the tissue radioactivity separated by thin layer chromatography on silica gel (chloroform/methanol/ammonia 18:6:1) in the heptane phase (*left*) and the aqueous phase (*right*) of the Dole extraction mixture of retinas incubated with [14C]palmitate. Most of the radioactivity incorporated into the phospholipids (bands in the lower half of plate) is discarded with the aqueous phase.

variation in its severity. Diabetic rat retina was found to produce significantly more $^{14}CO_2$ from [^{14}C]palmitate than normal retina; there were no major differences in other respects.

Three possible explanations occurred to us to account for the increased $^{14}CO_2$ production; first, that in diabetic retina, [^{14}C]palmitate entered a smaller oxidizable tissue pool; second, that the diabetic retina had an enhanced fat oxidizing capacity; and third, that increased oxidation of fat was a consequence of increased Krebs cycle activity. There is no evidence supporting the first possibility; on the contrary NEFA was not significantly less in diabetic rat retina (normal $2 \cdot 30 \pm 0 \cdot 29$ μequiv./g; diabetic $2 \cdot 12 \pm 0 \cdot 14$ μequiv./g) and, in alloxan diabetic rat heart, increased levels of fatty acyl CoA have been demonstrated (Garland, Randle and Newsholme, 1963). Bearing in mind the increased uptake of NEFA by the tissue at higher NEFA concentrations, an enhanced oxidative capacity of diabetic retina may be the adaptive sequel to the long raised circulating NEFA levels which characterize the diabetic state.

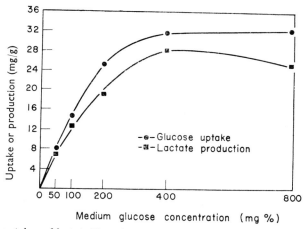

FIG. 13. Glucose uptake and lactate liberation into the incubation medium (measured enzymatically) expressed as mg/90 min per g wet wt of retina at various glucose concentrations. Glucose uptake (–●–●–); lactate production (–■–■–).

Chronic hyperglycaemia may also evoke adaptive changes in glucose metabolism, and evidence for such changes comes from several sources. Using histochemical techniques, Kurimoto and Newell (1963) demonstrated increased phosphorylase activity in diabetic rat retina and the augmented capacity of the diabetic retina for in vitro glycogen synthesis has been reported at this meeting (Kurimoto, Newell and Farkas, this Symposium). Illing and Gray (1951) showed that in the presence of pyruvate, retina from alloxan diabetic rabbits consumed more oxygen than the normal. De Roetth and Pei (1964) have also demonstrated greater oxygen consumption by retina from untreated diabetic rats stimulated by the presence of high concentrations of sodium succinate and glucose. The finding of supranormal levels of NAD and NADH in diabetic rat retina by Heath, Rutter and Beck (1962) would support the adaptation hypothesis, though it is difficult to reconcile this with their reported reduction in reduced NADP. Adaptive changes of this nature may occur elsewhere and quite rapidly, for Weber, Singhal and Srivastava (1964) have demonstrated increased enzyme synthesis in rat liver within a day or two of the induction of alloxan diabetes.

Can the subjection of retina to increased rates of glucose dissimilation in diabetes be linked in any way with the development of retinopathy? *In vitro,* as the concentration of glucose in the incubation medium rises, glucose uptake increases up to a limiting rate, and with it, lactate production (Fig. 13). In the presence of a raised blood sugar it is probable that the retina will be exposed to higher than normal concentrations not only of glucose but also of its metabolites. Figure 14 shows that for

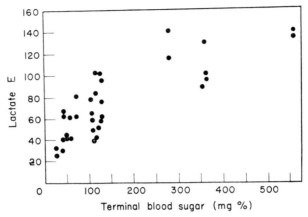

FIG. 14. The relationship between retinal tissue lactate concentration measured enzymatically and expressed as units of optical density (E) and the blood sugar measured at death (*abscissa*).

lactate this holds true. The retinal concentration of lactate measured within 30–60 sec of death shows a conspicuous rise as the terminal blood sugar increases. Variation in blood sugar was achieved by parenteral administration of glucose or insulin to normal and alloxanized rats.

The possible connection between raised concentrations of lactate and vascular changes in the retina has lately received increasing attention. The studies of Graymore (1964) and Graymore and Towlson (1963) of lactic acid dehydrogenase (LDH) levels in rat retina and the marked rise in fraction V of the enzyme during the vasoproliferative phase of experimental retrolental fibroplasia in the kitten point to a possible regulating role for lactate in vessel growth. Even more direct an indication is the recent claim of Imre (1964) to have induced intravitreal new vessel formation by injection of lactic acid into the vitreous body of the kitten. The clinical effect of salicylates on diabetic retinopathy may have an explanation along these lines. Not only may salicylate lower the blood sugar (Gilgore and Rupp, 1961) and hence the level of glucose at the retina, but the uncoupling effect of the ion (Smith, 1959; Whitehouse, 1964) may enhance the rate of oxidation of the products of glycolysis. Furthermore, it has been shown that LDH activity is inhibited by salicylate, perhaps further diminishing the local lactate concentration (Baker, 1960, 1961, 1962).

The effect of lactate on small blood vessels is disputed. De la Lande and Whelan (1962) seem to have disposed of the claim (Barcroft, and Cobbold, 1956) that the lactate ion acts as a vasodilator in exercising skeletal muscle. However, Veall (pers. comm.) has demonstrated, by means of radiosodium clearance, a vasodilatory effect of lactate in human skin. There may thus be regional differences in the vasomotor effects of lactate and it remains to be shown directly whether it affects the retinal vascular calibre in man. If so, high retinal lactate concentrations in the diabetic may explain the failure of a high partial pressure of oxygen to produce the vaso-constriction seen in the normal (Hickam and Sieker, 1960); it may also be the agent of the retinal venous dilatation described as the earliest visible retinal abnormality in the diabetic by many clinical observers. One may speculate too, about the effects of a prolonged vasodilator stimulus upon the pericyte or mural cell which probably controls capillary calibre, and the disappearance of which in the human diabetic retina antecedes the full development of retinopathy (Cogan and Kuwabara, 1963). The loss of capacity for capillary calibre adjustment in response to changing tissue requirements may lead to the shunt pattern described by Cogan with the dilated master capillary and the "dried-out" vascular bed about it. The apparent proliferation or possibly migration of capillary endothelial cells which accompanies the changes in the pericytes might also be interpreted as a response to the spurious 'anoxic' stimulus of high lactate concentration, spurious in that it results not from anoxia but from increased glycolysis.

Our present working hypothesis is that diabetic retinopathy may represent the retinal vascular response to long-standing increase in the local concentration of products of glucose catabolism, due to chronic hyperglycaemia. It would be naïve to suppose that this was a complete explanation. There has been strong advocacy of the views that retinopathy represents only a local manifestation of a generalized diabetic microangiopathy, that it results primarily from some abnormal constituent of the circulating blood or that it is the consequence of disturbed lipid or protein metabolism of the vessel wall itself; in addition, we have suggestive evidence that there may be circulating factors in diabetics which interfere with glucose metabolism in the retina, presumably at some insulin-insensitive step.

The attraction of this working hypothesis is its simplicity and its unifying nature; it has yet to be tested to destruction. Those with literary inclinations have dubbed the glucose lack of insulin-sensitive tissues in diabetes, "starvation in the midst of plenty". Is it too fanciful to suggest that as a direct consequence, the retina suffers from an embarras de richesses?

REFERENCES

Aarseth, S. (1953). *Acta med. scand. Suppl.* **281**, 146.

Ames, A. III and Gurian, B. S. (1963). *J. Neurophysiol.* **26**, 617.

Ashton, N. (1958). *Biblthca. ophthal. Basel* **8**, 1.

Ashton, N. (1959). *Lancet* **ii**, 625.

Baker, B. R. (1960). *J. mednl. pharm. Chem.* **2**, 633.

Baker, B. R. (1961). *J. Am. chem. Soc.* **83**, 3713.

Baker, B. R. (1962). *J. mednl. pharm. Chem.* **5**, 654.

Ballantyne, A. J. and Loewenstein, A. (1944). *Br. J. Ophthal.* **28**, 593.

Barcroft, H. and Cobbold, A. F. (1956). *J. Physiol. Lond.* **132**, 372.

Bastenie, P. A., Pirart, J. and Franckson, J. R. M. (1959). *Proceedings of the III Congress of the International Diabetes Federation.* Georg Thieme Verlag. Stuttgart.

Becker, B., Maengwyn-Davies, G. D., Rosen, D., Friedenwald, J. S. and Winter, F. C. (1954). *Diabetes* **3**, 175.

Bloodworth, J. M. B. (1962). *Diabetes* **11**, 1.

Blumenthal, H. T., Alex, M. and Goldenberg, S. (1961). *Am. J. Med.* **31**, 382.

Borgström, B. (1952). *Acta physiol. scand.* **25**, 101.

Brown, I. K. and Jones, A. T. (1964). *Br. J. Ophthal.* **48**, 148.

Caird, F. I. and Garratt, C. J. (1962). *Proc. R. Soc. Med.* **55**, 477.

Chlouverakis, C. and Keen, H. (1964). 'The Nature and Treatment of Diabetes Mellitus'. *Proceedings of the IV Congress of the International Diabetics Federation.* (To be Published).

Cogan, D. G. and Kuwabara, T. (1963). *Diabetes* **12**, 293.

Cogan, D. G., Toussaint, D. and Kuwabara, T. (1961). *Arch. Ophthal,* **66**, 366

Coleman, S. L., Becker, B., Canaan, S. and Rosenbaum, L. (1962). *Diabetes* **11**, 375.

De la Lande, I. S. and Whelan, R. F. (1962). *J. Physiol. Lond.* **162**, 151.

De Roetth, A. J. and Pei, Y. F. (1964). *Arch. Ophthal* **71**, 73.

Dole, V. P. (1956). *J. clin. Invest.* **35**, 150.

Dole, V. P. and Meinertz, H. (1960). *J. biol. Chem.* **235**, 2595.

Duncan, L. J. P., MacFarlane, A. and Robson, J. S. (1958). *Lancet* **i**, 822.

Dunlop, D. M. (1954). *Br. med. J.* **ii**, 383.

Engleson, G. (1954). *Studies in Diabetes Mellitus*, pp. 28–48. Berlingska Boktryckeriet.

Esmann, V., Jensen, H. J. and Lundbaek, K. (1963). *Acta med. scand.* **174**, 99.

Folch, J., Lees, M. and Stanley, J. H. S. (1957). *J. biol. Chem.* **226**, 497.

Garland, P. B., Randle, P. J. and Newsholme, E. A. (1963). *Nature Lond.* **200**, 169.

Gilgore, S. G. and Rupp, J. J. (1961). *Metabolism* **10**, 419.

Graymore, C. (1964). *Nature, Lond.* **201**, 615.

Graymore, C. N. and Towlson, M. (1963). *Exp. Eye Res.* **2**, 48.

Hardin, R. C., Jackson, R. L., Johnston, T. L. and Kelly, H. G. (1956) *Diabetes* **5**, 397.

Hausler, H. R., Sibay, T. M. and Campbell, J. (1964). *Diabetes* **13**, 123.

Heath, H., Rutter, A. C. and Beck, T. C., (1962). *Vision Res.* **2**, 333.

Hickam, J. B. and Sieker, H. O. (1960). *Circulation* **22**, 243.

Illing, E. K. B. and Gray, C. H., (1951). *J. Endocr.* **7**, 242.

Imre, G. (1964). *Br. J. Ophthal.* **48**, 75.

Johnsson, S. (1960). *Diabetes* **9**, 1.

Keen, H. and Chlouverakis, C. (1964). *Biochem. J.* (1965) **94**, 488.

Keen, H., Field, J. B. and Pastan, I. H. (1963). *Metabolism* **12**, 143.

Keen, H. and Smith, R. (1959). *Lancet* **i**, 849.

Kerpel, S., Shafrir, E. and Shapiro, B. (1961). *Biochim. biophys. Acta* **46**, 495.

Kurimoto, S. and Newell, F. W. (1963). *Invest. Ophthal.* **2**, 24.

Lancet, (1959). **ii**, 653, Leader.

Lawrence, R. D. (1949). *Lancet*, **ii**, 401.

Levene, R., Robertson, A. L., Foglia, V. G. and Singer, J. (1963). *Arch. Ophthal.* **70**, 253.

Lundbaek, K. (1953). 'Long Term Diabetes' Copenhagen.

Mooney, A. J. (1963). *Br. J. Ophthal.* **47**, 513.

Musacchio, I. T. L., Palermo, N. and Rodriguez, R. R. (1964). *Lancet* **i**, 146.

Pope, C. H. (1960). *Diabetes*, **9**, 9.

Powell, E. and Field, R. A. (1964). *Lancet*, **i**, 17.

Randle, P. J., Garland, P. B., Hales, C. N. and Newsholme, E. A. (1963). *Lancet* **i**, 785.

Schrade, W., Boehle, E., Biegler, R. and Harmuth, E. (1963). *Lancet* **i**, 285.

Scott, G. I. (1953). *Br. J. Ophthal.* **37**, 705.

Smith, M. J. H. (1959). *J. Pharm. Pharmacol* **11**, 705.

Umbreit, W. W., Burris, R. H. and Stauffer, J. F. (1964). 'Manometric Techniques'. Burgess Publishing Co. Minneapolis, Minn.

Weber, G., Singhal, R. L. and Srivastava, S. K. (1964). *Excerpta Med.* **74**, 58.

Werk, E. E. Jr. and Knowles, H. C. Jr. (1961). *Diabetes*, **10**, 22.

Whitehouse, M. W. (1964). *Biochem. Pharmac.* **13**, 319.

Woeller, F. H. (1961). *Analyt. Biochem.* **2**, 508.

DISCUSSION

Professor Ashton expressed enthusiasm for Dr. Keen's attempt to approach this complex field from a biochemical standpoint. The problem, he felt, lay in attempting to classify the nature of the disease. It was obviously vascular in manifestation, but one had to differentiate between such effects being primary or secondary in nature; if the former, then were these effects localized or generalized? Many people, he added, believed it to be a local manifestation of a general vascular disorder, and referred to it as diabetic microangiopathy. If that definition were correct, then why should one search for specific metabolic changes in the tissues themselves, rather than, for example, the endothelial cells of the vessel wall? There was abundant evidence to suggest that the endothelial cells of the retina were peculiar.

Dr. Keen's emphasis on the condition being secondary to environmental changes in the tissue was, nevertheless, of great interest to PROFESSOR ASHTON, as he had been the first to introduce the approach of examining the tissue *per se*. One vital factor, he felt, was that these changes were not specific, but that a variety of conditions might produce similar changes. One had to find the common pathway in the aetiology. PROFESSOR ASHTON finished his comments by asking Dr. Keen whether he had carried out any comparative studies on brain tissue, in which there was no evidence of vascular disturbances in even the most advanced stages of diabetes.

DR. KEEN explained that he had not personally examined brain tissue, but that the lower lactic acid production of this tissue might account for its differing reaction to diabetes.

PROFESSOR NOELL said that he had always been interested in the transfer of information between tissue and vessels, and was most interested in the localized nature of diabetic retinopathy. He questioned the possibility that light might be a contributory factor in the induction of such changes. His own work (reported in part at this meeting), suggested a potentially damaging effect of light on the visual cells, and one knew also, he pointed out, of the effects of light on skin, and the role of melanin in trapping light energy. He thought that one should not exclude the possibility that changes in diabetic retinopathy may be associated with light-energy effects on the endothelial cells.

PROFESSOR ASHTON, in reply to PROFESSOR NOELL, pointed out that there were certain objections to implicating light in the aetiology of diabetic retinopathy. The effect Professor Noell had described applied specifically to the visual cells, and these elements were not affected early in the course of the disease, nor was there any evidence for disturbances in the areas in which the visual cells lie. Furthermore, diabetic retinopathy continues to advance in the blind eye, and even in the cataractous eye.

PROFESSOR NEWELL preferred to view the condition as an ocular manifestation of a widespread disturbance of the vascular basement membrane. Electron microscopy of the diabetic kidney provided a very typical appearance suggesting a specific lesion in this organ. He also wished to remark on the curious phenomenom of patients showing all the ophthalmoscopic appearances of diabetic retinopathy, and on whom renal biopsy revealed characteristic basement membrane changes, and yet showed no chemical evidence of diabetes. Some 4–5 years later these patients developed the chemical signs of overt diabetes.

PROFESSOR ASHTON wished to point out that basement membrane thickening is not generalized; it had not, for example, been demonstrated in fat tissue and it had not been proved conclusively that it occurred in the retina. Bloodworth's work, of necessity, was carried on advanced post-mortem material, in which it is difficult to assess the significance of the thickening. Becker's demonstration of thickening in the basement membrane of the ciliary body had not been confirmed. Quite apart from these objections to a primary role of thickening in diabetic retinopathy, it is clear that thickening can occur in the absence of other diabetic changes. PROFESSOR ASHTON wondered, therefore, how these facts fitted into the pattern, and felt sure that other factors must be involved.

DR. HEATH expressed interest in Dr. Keen's hypothesis regarding the role of lactic acid in vasoproliferation, but doubted its significance on the grounds that his own alloxan diabetic rats had blood sugars ranging from 400–600 mg% yet they showed no vascular abnormalities. From what Dr. Keen had said, these high sugars should be associated with elevated levels of lactic acid.

DR. HEATH believed that rather than studying a variety of complex enzyme systems at random, one should look for the primary key in the process. He compared the situation to that of retrolental fibroplasia—if one had looked for the enzyme changes that followed the gross pathological changes it seems that this would have been of little avail as regards curing the condition. The simple key was oxygen, and one must search for a similar key in diabetic retinopathy. It was for this reason that his attention was now turning to the capillary wall. The vascular wall, he pointed out, is known to exhibit a high metabolic activity, including the active synthesis of lipoprotein and mucopolysaccharide. He suggested that an abnormal deposition of mucopolysaccharide within the walls might be involved, and these were the lines along which he was working.

PROFESSOR ASHTON agreed with Dr. Heath's analysis, but reminded him that changes in mucopolysaccharide could not be demonstrated in the early stages of the disease. One had yet to find the simple starting point.

DR. TOULSON said that she would like to mention results of work carried out conjointly with Dr. Graymore. They had found that insulin had no effect on glucose utilization of the retina. They had also measured the lactic acid content of the rapidly frozen retina taken from both alloxan and insulin treated animals and been unable to demonstrate any significant difference between these levels and those of the normal.

   Dr. Graymore and Dr. Towlson had measured pyridine nucleotide levels in the retina of the normal and alloxan-diabetic rat, and the results were essentially the same as those of Dr. Heath and his co-workers. It was of interest, however, that although insulin treatment of the normal animal reversed the ratio in the NAD system relative to the diabetic state, the change in the NADP system following insulin treatment was of the same sign as that of alloxan treatment. DR. TOWLSON also mentioned that they had been unable to confirm de Roetth's finding that anaerobic glycolysis was reduced in the alloxan diabetic rat.

MISS BROWN added that Dr. Graymore and she had also measured glucose uptake and lactic acid production of rat retinas incubated in serum from normal and diabetic patients, and shown some degree of inhibition in the latter.

The Retinal Vascular System in Experimental Diabetes*

A. C. RUTTER AND H. HEATH

Department of Chemical Pathology, University College Hospital Medical School, London, England

Endothelial proliferation, tortuosity and increases in PAS-positive material were found in the retinal veins from rats maintained in a severe state of diabetes for 145 days. The administration of β-aminopropionitrile to diabetic weanling rats gave similar results after 44 days. Treatment of diabetic rats with β,β'-iminodipropionitrile for 36 days, led to occlusion of the retinal arteries with PAS-positive material, but the capilaries and veins were not affected. Similar results were obtained on treating normal rats with β,β'-iminodipropionitrile and cortisol.

1. Introduction

The typical microaneurysms, characteristic of human diabetic retinopathy, are only occasionally observed in the retina of diabetic animals. There are some reports of retinal microaneurysms in experimental animals but these cases are exceptional and it is not possible for these lesions to be readily induced with certainty. Becker (1952) found that the administration of ACTH to the alloxan-diabetic rabbit led to the development of retinal microaneurysms but this observation has not been confirmed. Retinal microaneurysms were not observed when alloxan-diabetic rats were maintained on a high fat diet for 3 months (Kirschner and Leopold, 1960), but segmental thinning of the capillary reticulum occurred. Musacchio, Palermo and Rodriguez (1964) found dilatation of the arteries and veins, loss of transverse striations of the arteries, and arterial aneurysms in the retinas of rats, maintained for 3–7 months, following 95% pancreatectomy. In their studies on a Chinese hamster, Hausler, Sibay and Stachowska (1963) noted the appearance of several aneurysms of the capillaries and arterioles after 3 months of metahypophyseal diabetes. More recently, Hausler, Sibay and Campbell (1964) observed numerous capillary aneurysms in the retina of a metasomatotrophin-diabetic 10-year-old dog, but these aneurysms only developed after the dog had been diabetic for 8 years.

In previous communications, we have studied the activities of certain enzymes and the concentrations of coenzymes in the alloxan-diabetic rat retina in order that the biochemical changes responsible for the development of microaneurysms might be detected before the aneurysms appeared. It was considered, however, that an alternative approach to the problem of diabetic retinopathy would be an attempt to accelerate the rate of formation of retinal lesions in experimental animals. Abnormal deposits of PAS-positive hyaline material occur at the site of the microaneurysms in human diabetic retinopathy. Experiments have therefore been carried out in which alloxan-diabetic rats have been treated with β-aminopropionitrile, β,β'-iminodipropionitrile and cortisol. The administration of β-aminopropionitrile leads to the abnormal formation of intercellular ground substance, weakening of collagen fibres by inhibiting the formation of stable cross-linkages and eventual death from dissecting aneurysm of the aorta. The related compound, β,β'-iminodipropionitrile, has been observed by Selye (1957) to cause retinal haemorrhages especially in the cortisol-treated rat.

*This research was supported by grants from the Medical Research Council and the British Foundation for Research into the Prevention of Blindness.

2. Experimental

Animals

Weanling (50 g) or young (100–200 g) albino male rats were used and fed on MRC diet 41 *ad lib.* Weanling and young rats were made diabetic by the alloxan injection method of Klebanoff and Greenbaum (1954) and the high mortality rate of weanling rats was partially overcome by giving each rat a daily injection of 1 unit of insulin Zinc Suspension, B.P. ("Lente") for 1 week after the alloxan injection.

β-Aminopropionitrile (BAPN), β,β'-iminodipropionitrile (IDPN) and cortisol were given by mouth and in order to obtain a more continuous and prolonged effect, these were added as solutions to the drinking water to give the following approximate daily dose levels: BAPN, 100 mg/100 g body weight; IDPN, 30 mg/100 g body weight, and cortisol, 1 mg/100 g body weight.

Blood glucose

Blood glucose was determined by the glucose oxidase method of Huggett and Nixon (1957) on 0·025 ml of tail vein blood, or by the *o*-toluidine method of Hultman (1959) as modified by Hyvärinen and Nikkilä (1962), on 0·05 ml of tail vein blood. Polyuria and hyperglycaemia (greater than 200 mg glucose/100 ml blood) were taken as indications of diabetes.

Retinal preparations

The rats were killed by cervical dislocation and the eyes fixed in formol-saline for at least 48 hr before further treatment. Flat retinal vascular system preparations were made by the tryptic digestion method of Kuwabara and Cogan (1960). The digested rat retina was extremely difficult to handle since it readily became entangled. Debris was removed from the partially digested retina by aspirating it several times into a 0·8 mm bore capillator tube. When digestion was complete, the vascular tree was transfered by means of the capillator tube to a slide for mounting. This was conveniently carried out by placing a perspex ring, 18 mm internal diameter and 4 mm deep, on the slide and filling the cavity with 10% ethanol. After the vascular tree had been arranged in the desired position on the surface, with fine forceps, the 10% ethanol was withdrawn from under the ring with the aid of absorbent tissue, thus allowing the retinal vascular system to remain flat. After all the 10% ethanol was removed, the preparation was dried and stained with periodic acid-Schiff (PAS) and haematoxylin.

3. Results

The eight retinas from the eyes of four alloxan-diabetic rats, maintained in a state of severe diabetes for 145 days, all showed marked pathological changes. These were most apparent in the branch veins (Plate 1) which were tortuous and contained more PAS-positive material in the walls. Many of the branch veins still contained erythrocytes although these were not present in retinal preparations from normal rats (Plate 2). Endothelial proliferation could also be observed in these branch veins. In one retina, some branch arteries were dilated (Plate 3). No pathological changes could be observed in the capillaries. In a control series of rats which had been injected with alloxan but had not developed diabetes, the retinal vascular system was normal.

Two alloxan-diabetic weanling rats, treated with BAPN, were found to have tortuous retinal branch veins, with increased PAS-positive material and endothelial proliferation (Plate 4), after 56 and 62 days, although no signs of pathological changes could be detected in the retinas from two rats similarly treated for 11 and 55 days.

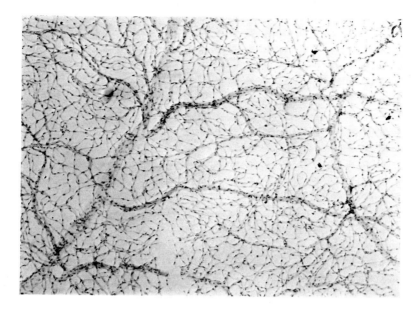

PLATE 1. Part of the retinal vascular system from a 145-day-diabetic rat showing increased PAS-positive material and endothelial proliferation in tortuous branch veins. (× 70)

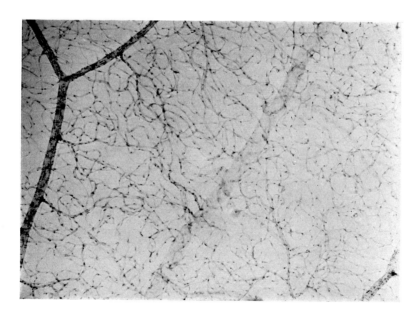

PLATE 2. Part of the normal retinal vascular system from an adult rat. (× 70)

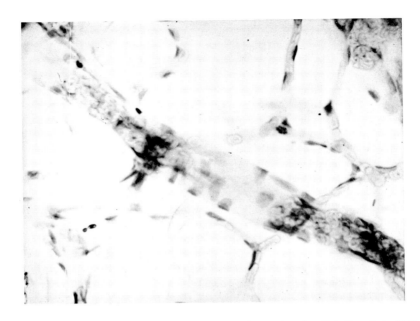

PLATE 3. Fusiform dilatation of a retinal artery from a 145-day-diabetic rat. ($\times$550)

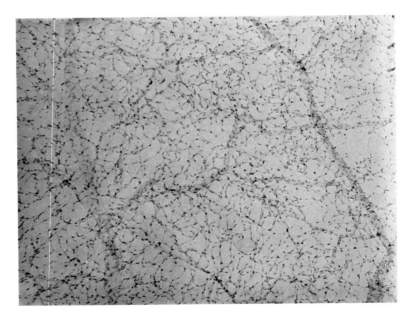

PLATE 4. Part of the retinal vascular system from a 62-day-β-aminopropionitrile-treated diabetic rat showing increased PAS-positive material and endothelial proliferation in a tortuous branch vein. ($\times$ 70)

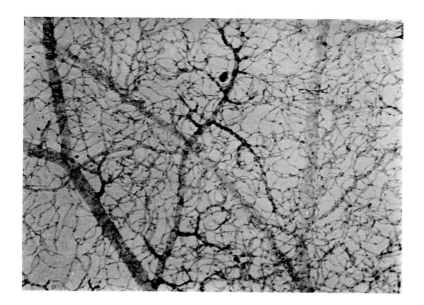

PLATE 5. Part of the retinal vascular system from a 36-day-β,β'-iminodipropionitrile-treated diabetic rat showing deposition of PAS-positive material and occlusion of branch arteries. (× 70)

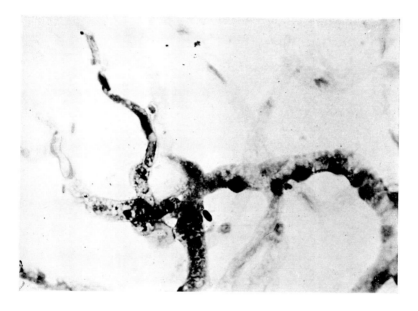

PLATE 6. Deposits of PAS-positive material and occlusion in a retinal branch artery from a 36-day-β,β'-iminodipropionitrile-treated diabetic rat. (× 550)

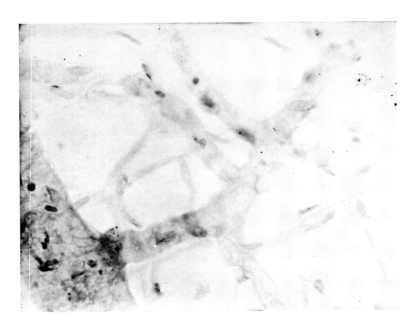

PLATE 7. Deposits of PAS-positive material in a retinal branch artery from a 42-day-β,β'-iminodi-propionitrile-treated rat. ($\times$ 550)

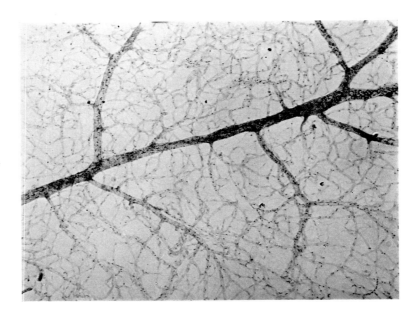

PLATE 8. Part of the retinal vascular system from a 42-day-β,β'-iminodipropionitrile-treated rat showing PAS-positive fusiform dilatations of a main artery and loss of transverse striation. ($\times$ 70)

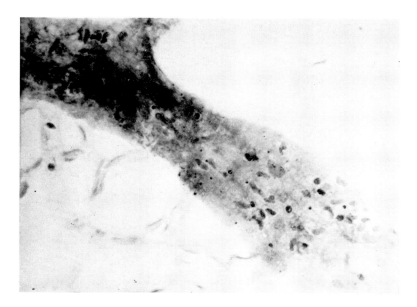

PLATE 9. Dilatation of a retinal artery from a 42-day-β,β'-iminodipropionitrile-treated rat showing loss of transverse striation and deposition of PAS-positive material. ($\times$ 550)

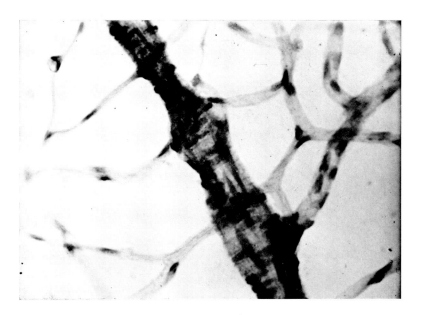

PLATE 10. Fusiform dilatations of a retinal artery from a 14-day-β,β'-iminodipropionitrile and cortisol-treated diabetic rat. ($\times$ 550)

The retinas from 5 weanling rats treated with BAPN alone for up to 64 days were found to be normal.

Treatment of young alloxan-diabetic rats with IDPN for periods up to 36 days led to the heavy deposition of PAS-positive material in the retinal branch arteries, initially in the position of the mural cells, and in some cases to such an extent as to cause complete occlusion (Plates 5 and 6). There were, however, no changes in either the veins or capillaries. When IDPN was administered to young normal rats for periods up to 49 days, increases in the content of PAS-positive material in the retinal branch arteries were also observed (Plate 7), although to a lesser extent than those occurring in the IDPN-treated diabetic animals and there were no apparent arterial occlusions. No changes in the structure of the capillaries and veins could be seen, but extensive PAS-positive fusiform dilatations of the main arteries were present, with loss of transverse striations (Plates 8 and 9).

4. Discussion

The maintenance of young rats in a severe state of uncontrolled diabetes for periods from 3–6 months does lead to the development of pathological changes in the retinal vascular system. That these changes are due to the diabetes and not to the treatment with alloxan, has been established by the fact that the alloxan-injected rats which did not develop diabetes, had normal retinal vascular systems. Although increased deposition of PAS-positive material occurred in the retinal branch veins of the alloxan-diabetic animals, no microaneurysms were observable and the diabetic animals were therefore treated with BAPN and IDPN so as to accelerate the deposition of PAS-positive material in the hope that the formation of microaneurysms might be induced.

Selye (1957) has reported that the administration of IDPN to rats and other species leads to the development of corneal opacities, intra-ocular haemorrhages and retinal detachment. We have observed that the administration of IDPN to normal rats brings about the deposition of large amounts of PAS-positive material in the retinal arteries. When this compound was fed to the diabetic animals, this deposition was even more marked and numerous arterial occlusions were observed. The localization of this effect in the arteries was unexpected and no abnormal deposits took place in either the veins or capillaries. One retina was found to be deeply detached in the eye of a diabetic animal after 36 days of IDPN treatment. Selye has reported that the simultaneous administration of cortisol with IDPN leads to exacerbation of the ocular effects, which we too have observed. Numerous retinal arteries were occluded in preparations from normal rats after 48 days of cortisol and IDPN treatment but the veins and capillaries were still unaffected. Attempts to maintain alloxan-diabetic rats on cortisol and IDPN were unsuccesful since the three animals so treated only survived for 9, 14 and 16 days. By that time, deposits of PAS-positive material had not occurred and the only observable pathological change was a fusiform dilatation of a retinal branch artery (Plate 10).

The effects of administering BAPN to young rats differed markedly from those brought about by the related compound, IDPN. Young rats, treated with BAPN for 44 days, although exhibiting signs of osteolathyrism such as bone malformation of the hind legs, did not have any abnormal deposition of PAS-positive material or any abnormality in the retinal vasculature. BAPN has a greater effect on the aorta when administered to weanling rats (Schmidt and Orbison, 1962) and it was decided to determine whether this compound would affect the retinal vascular system if administration was commenced as soon as the animals had been weaned. Even though the osteolathyritic symptoms which developed were more severe and at least one animal died of aortic rupture, there were still no observable changes in the retina after 46 days' treatment with this compound. In the retinas from two alloxan-diabetic rats, which had been made diabetic immediately after weaning and maintained on BAPN for 56 and 62 days, there were signs of endothelial proliferation and increased PAS staining, in addition to tortuosity of the veins. No abnormalities in the capillaries or arteries were observed in animals treated with BAPN. Attempts to study the effect of cortisol superimposed upon the BAPN treatment of the normal and alloxan-diabetic weanling rats could not be successfully completed, owing to the high toxicity of this combination of drugs.

Retinal microaneurysms do not always occur in human diabetics and it may be possible that in those patients in which diabetic retinopathy is a serious complication, there is some other metabolic defect which enhances the deposition of PAS-positive chondromucoprotein in the retinal capillaries. The fact that diabetic rats do not develop these lesions even when suffering from uncontrolled diabetes for a considerable length of time, may indicate that some other stress or metabolic defect might have to be superimposed on the diabetes, if experimental animals with the characteristic lesions of human diabetic retinopathy are to be obtained. The effects of two toxic compounds, both of which derange glycosaminoglycan metabolism, have been studied but in neither case has this resulted in the appearance of capillary microaneurysms. IDPN, however, did exert a severe toxic effect on the retina, resulting in arterial occlusion and retinal detachment. There are many other compounds, some of which are structurally related to the aminonitriles (Ressler, Redstone and Erenberg, 1961), having lathyrogenic effects. Some of these occur naturally in vegetable materials (Bell, 1964) and α, γ-diaminobutyric acid has also been reported to occur in bovine liver (Ackermann and Menssen, 1960). The effects of these compounds and their possible occurrence in diabetic tissues is being investigated.

ACKNOWLEDGMENTS

We wish to thank Professor Norman Ashton and Miss A. Arrowsmith for their help and Abbott Laboratories Ltd. for their generous gift of β-aminopropionitrile.

REFERENCES

Ackermann, D. and Menssen, H. G. (1960). *Z. Physiol. Chem.* **318**, 212.
Becker, B. (1952). *Ann. intern. Med.* **37**, 273.
Bell, E. A. (1964). *Nature, Lond.* **203**, 378.
Hausler, H. R., Sibay, T. M. and Campbell, J. (1964). *Diabetes* **13**, 122.
Hausler, H. R., Sibay, T. M. and Stachowska, B. (1963). *Am. J. Ophthal.* **56**, 242.
Huggett, A. St. G. and Nixon, D. A. (1957). *Lancet* **ii**, 368.
Hultman, E. (1959). *Nature, Lond.* **183**, 108.
Hyvärinen, A. and Nikkilä, E. A. (1962). *Clinica chim. Acta* **7**, 140.
Kirschner, R. and Leopold, I. H. (1960). *Arch. Ophthal.* **64**, 681.
Klebanoff, S. J. and Greenbaum, A. L. (1954). *J. Endocr.* **11**, 311.
Kuwabara, T. and Cogan, D. (1960). *Arch. Ophthal.* **64**, 904.
Musacchio, I. T. L., Palermo, N. and Rodriguez, R. R. (1964). *Lancet* **i**, 146.
Ressler, C., Redstone, P. A. and Erenberg, R. H. (1961). *Science* **134**, 188.
Schmidt, G. and Orbison, J. L. (1962). *Fed. Proc.* **21**, 168.
Selye, H. (1957). *Revue can. Biol.* **16**, 1.

The Glycosaminoglycans of the Normal and Alloxan-diabetic Rat Retina and Aorta

R. A. PATERSON AND H. HEATH

Department of Chemical Pathology, University College Hospital Medical School, London, England

The quantitative separation and determination of the hyaluronic acid, chondroitin sulphate, heparin and neutral glycosaminoglycans from the normal and alloxan-diabetic rat retina and aorta showed that there were significant decreases in the chondroitin sulphate content in both tissues and in the content of the neutral glyco-saminoglycan fraction of the retina in the diabetic state. In agreement with this observed diminished chondroitin sulphate content, *in vitro* incorporation of $^{35}SO_4$ into the glycosaminoglycans of the aorta was reduced in alloxan-diabetes and un-affected by insulin *in vitro*. The administration of insulin *in vivo* did not significantly alter the uptake of $^{35}SO_4$, but caused a decrease in the quantity incorporated into the glycosaminoglycan fraction.

1. Introduction

Deposits of hyaline material are known to occur at the site of microaneurysms in human diabetic retinopathy and Toussaint, Cogan and Kuwabara (1962) observed that the number of deposits increased with the severity of the capillary lesions. Anderson (1963) has shown that the precipitates formed from certain plasma proteins and chondroitin sulphate are similar to pathological deposits of hyaline material. Curran (1957) has demonstrated that the endothelium of vascular tissue is a major site for chondroitin sulphate biosynthesis. Abnormalities in the rate of formation of sulphated glycosaminoglycans (GAG) by diabetic vascular endothelium may lead to abnormal deposition of hyaline-like chondromucoproteins. It was therefore decided to investigate the rate of formation of chondroitin sulphate and to determine the quantities of hyaluronic acid, chondroitin sulphate, heparin and the neutral GAG in the alloxan-diabetic rat retina and aorta.

2. Methods

Male albino rats, 150–200 g, maintained on MRC diet 41 *ad lib.*, were made diabetic by the subcutaneous injection of alloxan (Klebanoff and Greenbaum, 1954). Blood glucose was determined on 25 μl tail vein blood by the glucose oxidase method (Huggett and Nixon, 1957) or on 50 μl by the *o*-toluidine method of Hultman (1959) as modified by Hyvärinen and Nikkilä (1962). The diabetic animals had blood glucose levels between 200 and 500 mg/100 ml and were sacrificed between 3 and 8 weeks after injection.

Quantitative estimation of glycosaminoglycans

The GAG contents of normal and alloxan-diabetic aorta and retina were estimated by a modification of the method of Antonopoulos, Gardell, Szirmai and de Tyssonsk (1964). The eyes were enucleated, incised equatorially and the cornea, lens and vitreous humour removed. The retina was carefully separated from the sclera and choroid under 0·9% NaCl and the excess saline was absorbed with filter paper. The aorta was excised and the connective tissue removed. One aorta or two retinas were suspended in 0·2 ml digestion medium so as to give between 1 and 2 mg wet tissue/10 μl digest. The medium consisted of 0·1 M phosphate buffer, pH 6·5, containing 5 mM EDTA, 5 mM cysteine HCl, 5 mM

*This research was supported by grants from the Medical Research Council and the British Foundation for Research into the Prevention of Blindness.

Na_2SO_4 and 0·25 mg crystalline papain/ml. The tissues were digested for 18 hr at 65°C and the digest was applied to a column (60 × 3 mm) of cellulose powder (0·1 g) previously washed with 5 ml 1% cetyl pyridinium chloride (CPC). One ml 1% CPC was passed through the column and hyaluronic acid, chondroitin sulphate and heparin were eluted with 1ml 0·5 M NaCl, 0·7 M $MgCl_2$ and 1·25 M $MgCl_2$, respectively, all containing 0·05% CPC. Any remaining complex was dissolved with 1 ml 6 N HCl.

The GAG in the fractions containing $MgCl_2$ were precipitated by the addition of 0·5 ml 1% CPC and 3 ml water and collected by centrifugation, since these concentrations of $MgCl_2$ interfere with the subsequent estimation.

After hydrolysis for 8 hr in 6 N HCl at 100°C, all fractions were estimated for hexosamine by the modified Elson and Morgan (1933) procedure, adapted by Antonopoulos et al (1964). The sensitivity of the method was increased by using a Unicam Spectrophotometer (Model S.P. 700) with cells of 4 cm light path.

Incorporation of $^{35}SO_4$

The effect of insulin on the incorporation of $^{35}SO_4$ by the isolated aorta was studied *in vitro* by the addition of 0·1 i.u. insulin (soluble)/ml incubation medium, and *in vivo* by the injection of 2 units insulin Zinc Suspension, B.P. ("Lente"), 2 units ("Lente") and 3 units (soluble) at 24-hr-intervals. The animals were maintained in metabolism cages and killed by cervical dislocation 1·5 hr after the last dose, if polyuria had ceased. Blood sugars were determined just before death.

Each thoracic aorta was incised longitudinally, stripped of connective tissue, washed in Krebs-Ringer phosphate solution, weighed and incubated at 37°C, with shaking, in 1 ml Krebs-Ringer solution. After 15 min, a solution (10^6 cts/min) of carrier-free $Na_2{}^{35}SO_4$ (Radiochemical Centre, Amersham) was added to each flask and incubated for 3 hr. Sodium iodoacetate (5 mM, final concentration) was then added and after a further 15 min incubation, the sections of aorta were washed with 3 × 1 ml 0·9% NaCl. After digesting the aortas as described above, the digest was cooled to 4°C, adjusted to pH 1·5 by the addition of HCl and the precipitated nucleic acids and proteins removed by centrifugation at 10,000 g for 10 min. The radioactivity of the supernatant was determined in duplicate on 20 µl aliquots. The GAG were precipitated by the addition of 0·25 ml 0·01 M Na_2SO_4 which aids the coagulation and precipitation of the complex (Scott, 1960) and 4·5 ml 3% Rivanol (Boström, Moretti and Whitehouse, 1963) and after standing for 30 hr at 4°C, removed by centrifugation at 25,000 g for 20 min. The radioactivity of the supernatant was determined in duplicate on 0·2 ml aliquots. The incorporation of $^{35}SO_4$ by the GAG/g of wet tissue was calculated by difference.

3. Results

The results of the quantitative determination of the neutral and acidic GAG in the normal and diabetic rat retina and aorta are given in Table I.

TABLE I

Glycosaminoglycan content of the normal and diabetic
rat retina and aorta

Tissue	Glycosaminoglycans µg hexosamine/g wet wt*			
	Neutral	Hyaluronic acid	Chondroitin sulphate	Heparin
Normal aorta (6)	1469 ± 113	245 ± 31	645 ± 61	89 ± 14
Diabetic aorta (5)	1520 ± 102	206 ± 25	430 ± 42	75 ± 10
Normal retina (6)	889 ± 96	197 ± 23	84 ± 12	42 ± 19
Diabetic retina (4)	648 ± 74	156 ± 46	42 ± 6	14 ± 11

* Results are expressed as the arithmetic mean ± S.E.M. The figures in parenthesis represent the number of animals.

The mean value for the chondroitin sulphate fraction of 645 ± 61 μg hexosamine/g wet weight of normal aorta differed significantly ($P<0{\cdot}02$) from the value of 430 ± 42 μg hexosamine/g wet weight of diabetic aorta. There were no significant differences between the hexosamine contents of the other GAG fractions. A similar decrease in the chondroitin sulphate content occurred in the diabetic rat retina. The difference was significant ($P<0{\cdot}02$) between the mean value of 84 ± 12 and 42 ± 6 μg hexosamine/g wet weight for the normal and diabetic retinas, respectively. There was also a significant difference ($P<0{\cdot}05$) between the normal (889 ± 96) and diabetic (648 ± 74 μg hexosamine/g wet weight) retinal neutral GAG. The low level of heparin in the retina was only just within the limits of accurate determination.

The percentage of the total hexosamine present in the chondroitin sulphate fractions from these tissues are given in Table II.

TABLE II

Percentages of the total hexosamine present in the chondroitin sulphate fractions from normal and diabetic rat retina and aorta

Tissue	No. of animals	Percentages*
Normal aorta	6	27·1 ± 2·4
Diabetic aorta	5	19·4 ± 0·7
Normal retina	6	7·2 ± 0·6
Diabetic retina	4	5·5 ± 0·8

* Results are expressed as the arithmetic mean ± S.E.M.

The proportion of the total hexosamine content of the retina present as chondroitin sulphate was considerably less than that in the aorta. There was a significant difference ($P<0{\cdot}005$) between the percentage of hexosamine present as chondroitin sulphate in the normal (27·1 ± 2·4) and the diabetic (19·4 ± 0·7) rat aorta. A decrease from 7·2 ± 0·6% to 5·5 ± 0·8% was observed for the corresponding fractions in the retina.

The effects of alloxan diabetes on the incorporation of $^{35}SO_4$ by the aorta are given in Table III.

TABLE III

The uptake of $^{35}SO_4$ and incorporation in glycosaminoglycans by aortas from normal and alloxan-diabetic rats

Animals	Blood glucose (mg/100 ml)*	$^{35}SO_4$ uptake (cts/min × 10⁻²) per g aorta		GAG as per cent of total*
		Total uptake*	GAG incorporation*	
Normal (7)	99 ± 4	1625 ± 215	1330 ± 295	80·0 ± 3·8
Diabetic (7)	358 ± 38	916 ± 150	740 ± 149	78·6 ± 3·3
Diabetic plus insulin *in vitro* (5)	373 ± 43	890 ± 180	698 ± 183	74·6 ± 4·4
Diabetic plus insulin *in vivo* (5)	61 ± 2	776 ± 206	438 ± 134	48·7 ± 10·3

* Results are expressed as the arithmetic mean ± S.E.M. The figures in parenthesis represent the number of animals.

There was a statistically significant decrease ($P<0.01$) in the rate of sulphate uptake by the normal and diabetic rat aorta. Neither the presence of insulin *in vitro*, nor the *in vivo* administration of insulin for at least 48 hr before the removal of the aorta, caused any increase in $^{35}SO_4$ uptake by the tissue from the diabetic animals. There were also significant decreases in the amount of sulphate incorporated into the GAG fraction between the normal and diabetic rat aorta ($P<0.02$) and between the aorta from the normal and diabetic rats previously treated with insulin *in vivo* ($P<0.005$). The percentages of the total sulphate incorporated into the GAG fraction were similar in the normal, diabetic and *in vitro* insulin-treated diabetic aorta, but there was a significant decrease ($P<0.005$) in the percentage incorporated by tissues from the diabetic animals previously treated with insulin *in vivo*.

4. Discussion

At the time of commencing this research, methods for the quantitative determination of the individual glycosaminoglycans in the isolated rat retinal vascular system were not available. It was therefore decided to determine the total content of hyaluronic acid, chondroitin sulphate and heparin in the retinas from both normal and diabetic animals and to compare these results with those obtained from similar determinations on the aorta. In alloxan-diabetes we have found that there are significant decreases in the chondroitin sulphate content of both the rat aorta and retina. In the former tissue there are no changes in the amounts of the other GAG in the neutral, hyaluronic acid and heparin fractions and it would seem that the derangement in GAG metabolism is associated only with the chondroitin sulphate fraction in the aorta of the alloxan-diabetic rat.

This decrease in the chondroitin sulphate content of the diabetic rat aorta is in agreement with the lower rate of $^{35}SO_4$ incorporation by this tissue. Schiller and Dorfman (1957) have observed reduced rates of GAG biosynthesis in the skin from alloxan-diabetic rats and Urritia, Beavan and Cahill (1962) and Mulcahy and Winegrad (1962) have reported that the *in vitro* incorporation of labelled glucose into the aortas of alloxan-diabetic rats was impaired, and unaffected by insulin *in vitro*, or pretreatment with insulin *in vivo*.

Picard, Gardais and Laccord (1962) have shown that considerable amounts of $^{35}SO_4$ are present as UDP-N-acetylgalectosamine sulphate in normal rat aorta, after *in vitro* incubation with radioactive sulphate. In their work the radioactivity showed a peak after 6 hr in this nucleotide fraction and a maximum after 24 hr in the GAG fraction. Dorfman (1963) reported a turnover for chondroitin sulphate of 7–10 days. In our experiments we found that up to 30% of the total uptake of $^{35}SO_4$ was incorporated into the non-GAG fraction after 3 hrs' incubation *in vitro* in normal and diabetic animals, with or without insulin *in vitro*. After pretreating the diabetic animals with insulin *in vivo*, 50% of the total uptake was incorporated into the non-GAG fraction. In these animals, the insulin caused marked hypoglycaemia and this may have been responsible for the failure to form fully polymerized GAG.

We have also found a significant decrease in the content of the neutral GAG fraction in the diabetic rat retina. In a preliminary communication Wortman and Freeman (1962) have reported that the bovine retina contains one non-sulphated and two sulphated acid GAG and one non-sulphated neutral GAG. Antonopoulos, Borelius, Gardell, Hamström and Scott (1961) have shown that the CPC-kerato-sulphate complex is soluble in 1% cetyl pyridinium chloride and will therefore not be retained by the CPC-treated cellulose column and, if present, would appear in the neutral fraction. The possibility therefore exists that the decrease found in the neutral fraction may reflect an alteration in keratosulphate metabolism. The micro-methods described above have made possible the separation of some of the individual glycosaminoglycans and work is still in progress on the determination of the rates of $^{35}SO_4$ incorporation into the retinal GAG fractions.

ACKNOWLEDGMENTS

We wish to thank Miss A. Arrowsmith for her assistance and Bayer Products Ltd. for their generous gift of Rivanol (Ethodin).

REFERENCES

Anderson, A. J. (1963). *Biochem. J.* **88**, 460.
Antonopoulos, C. A., Borelius, E., Gardell, S., Hamström, B. and Scott, J. E. (1961). *Biochim. biophys. Acta* **54**, 213.
Antonopoulos, C. A., Gardell, S., Szirmai, J. A. and de Tyssonsk, E. R. (1964). *Biochim. biophys. Acta* **83**, 1.
Boström, H., Moretti, A. and Whitehouse, M. W. (1963). *Biochim. biophys. Acta* **74**, 213.
Curran, R. C. (1957). *J. Path. Bact.* **74**, 347.
Dorfman, A. (1963). *J. Histochem. Cytochem.* **11**, 2.
Elson, L. A. and Morgan, W. T. J. (1933). *Biochem. J.* **27**, 1824.
Huggett, A. St. G. and Nixon, D. A. (1957). *Lancet* **ii**, 368.
Hultman, E. (1959). *Nature, Lond.* **183**, 108.
Hyvärinen, A. and Nikkilä, E. A. (1962). *Clinica chim. Acta* **7**, 140.
Klebanoff, S. J. and Greenbaum, A. L. (1954). *J. Endocr.* **11**, 311.
Mulcahy, P. D. and Winegrad, A. I. (1962). *Am. J. Physiol.* **203**, 1038.
Picard, J., Gardais, A. and Laccord, M. (1962). *C. r. hebd. Séanc. Acad. Sci., Paris* **225**, 2182.
Schiller, S. and Dorfman, A. (1957). *J. biol. Chem.* **227**, 625.
Scott, J. E. (1960). *Meth. of Biochem. Analysis* **8**, 145.
Toussaint, D., Cogan, D. G. and Kuwabara, T. (1962). *Arch. Ophthal.* **67**, 42.
Urritia, G., Beaven, D. W. and Cahill, G. F. (1962). *Metabolism* **11**, 530.
Wortman, B. and Freeman, M. (1962). *Fed. Proc.* **21**, 170.

DISCUSSION

DR. KEEN thought that one should consider the possibility that the reduction in the incorporation of ^{35}S in the aorta of the diabetic animal might result merely from the poor condition of the treated animals rather than the diabetes *per se*.

PROFESSOR ASHTON was very interested in the finding by Mr. Rutter that the mucopolysaccharide was deposited on the arterial side of the circulation, for this was seen also in hypertensive retinopathy. He suggested that in view of this it might be as well to check the effects of BAPN and IDPN on the blood pressure of the rats under investigation. PROFESSOR ASHTON also expressed great interest in the fact that occlusion, or narrowing of the artery, which was one of the suggested mechanisms of diabetic retinopathy, did not in fact lead in the experiments demonstrated to the changes typical of this condition. Dr. Henkind and he had produced complete obstruction of retinal arterioles by introduction of glass ballotini into experimental animals *via* the carotid route. Micro-aneurysms did not result from this treatment, so one was forced to conclude that factors other than simple arterial occlusion were involved in the pathogenesis of diabetic retinopathy. Professor Ashton continued by stressing once again that the changes in mucopolysaccharide should not be considered as specific, as such changes occurred in all micro-aneurysms, regardless of cause. He quoted sickle cell anaemia and hypertension as examples. Conversely, he cited a number of instances, including tuberculosis, carcinomatosis and pregnancy, in which there were disturbances in circulatory mucopolysaccharides without accompanying retinopathy.

DR. HENKIND emphasized the problem of artefact production when employing the digestion technique—this was particularly applicable to the demonstration of arterial dilatations. On the advice of Professor Ashton, he was now combining the digest and injection techniques in order to obtain a more realistic overall picture of the vascular architecture. Certain disparities had been revealed by use of these methods, although he felt it was too early to assess the significance of these differences at this stage.

DR. KUWABARA congratulated Mr. Rutter on the excellence of his pictures and said that he was particularly impressed that these changes had been found as early as 140 days after treatment, as Dr. Bloodworth and he had formed the impression that it took some 4 years for such changes to develop and become apparent. Nevertheless, he felt convinced that the changes were characteristic of diabetes. He showed the meeting a preparation from his colony of Chinese hamsters. These animals had been shown to develop a spontaneous diabetes, and his opinion was that the earliest change involved a loss of muscle cells from the vessel wall.

PROFESSOR ASHTON challenged Dr. Kuwabara's suggestion that his own pictures were identical to those obtained by Mr. Rutter, and pointed out that Dr. Kuwabara's slide showed capillary closure and aneurysm formation, thus presenting an entirely different situation. DR. KUWABARA explained that he was limiting his comparison to dilatation effects. DR. HENKIND then showed the meeting the picture resulting from the experimental occlusion he had described, and suggested that this was also identical to that shown by Dr. Kuwabara except that once again there was no aneurysm formation. He said that he and Professor Ashton had shown that such capillary changes, the formation of the so-called preferential beds, could occur within 13 days of the occlusion, and he agreed with Professor Ashton that such changes probably had nothing to do with diabetes.

DR. HEATH doubted if the changes demonstrated could be attributed to artefacts on the grounds that such changes were not evident in the controls. PROFESSOR ASHTON agreed that the number of controls endorsed the validity of the findings.

DR. KEEN asked whether any member of the meeting was familiar with Byrom's technique for the direct viewing of the retina. PROFESSOR ASHTON said his department employed this procedure quite routinely in studies on hypertension, but that they had not so far turned its use to diabetic retinopathy, which was extremely difficult to produce experimentally.

The Effect of Sodium Ions on Glucose Metabolism of Ciliary Body and Retina

M. V. Riley

Institute of Ophthalmology, University of London, England

Measurements were made on the rates of glycolysis and respiration of retina and ciliary body in media containing no sodium ions or including ouabain, an inhibitor of active sodium transport. Significant inhibition of oxygen uptake, glucose utilization and lactate production was found in both tissues. Under anaerobic conditions similar inhibition of glycolysis was apparent. Aerobically, a greater fraction of the glucose utilized was metabolized via the hexose monophosphate pathway.

These experiments, and the partial relief of inhibition by dinitrophenol, point to a regulatory role of Na-K-stimulated ATPase in carbohydrate metabolism by the control of ADP levels available for oxidative phosphorylation and the phosphokinases of the Embden-Meyerhof pathway.

The significance of the unusually high glycolytic rate in ciliary body was discussed.

1. Introduction

The function of both ciliary body and retina is concerned with the movement of sodium ions across cell membranes, in the former as the initial process in the formation of aqueous humour, and in the latter to establish polarized membrane potentials for the transmission of nervous impulses. These two tissues have the same embryonic origin and, in spite of their very different specialization during development, in the adult eye they are found to have certain similar characteristics in their metabolism and, in fact, are unique among normal animal tissues in having a high rate of aerobic glycolysis. The present paper deals with the relationship between ion transport in these tissues and the metabolic processes which generate the required energy.

The role of Na-K-stimulated ATPase in the active transport of sodium and potassium ions has been widely investigated during the last 5 years (Skou, 1960; Bonting, Simon and Hawkins, 1961), and it is apparent that transport of sodium across a cell membrane or cell layer, against an electrochemical gradient, is closely geared to the hydrolysis of ATP and consequently, is dependent upon energy yielding mechanisms. Inhibition of respiration by cyanide or an anaerobic atmosphere inhibits the formation of aqueous humour, and dinitrophenol produces the same effect (Cole, 1961). Transport of sodium is similarly affected in brain and kidney under conditions which prevent the formation of high energy bonds by oxidative phosphorylation, whereas in erythrocytes the sodium pump is dependent upon glycolytically produced ATP and is insensitive to cyanide or uncouplers, as aerobic metabolism is of little significance in these cells.

It has recently been shown that in brain and kidney the oxidative activity of the tissues is partly controlled by the activity of the sodium transporting mechanism (Whittam and Blond, 1964; Whittam and Willis, 1963). Inhibition of the sodium pump by ouabain causes a fall in the oxygen uptake of the tissue, indicating that the

149

ADP levels which regulate the rate of electron transport are determined in part by the activity of the Na-K ATPase.

2. Methods

Pig eyes were obtained from freshly killed animals and transported in crushed ice. All operations were then carried out on ice and the tissues were ready for incubation within 5 hr of death. The ciliary body and iris were removed from the anterior segment and then the iris and most of the posterior part of the ciliary body were cut away, leaving a thin circle of tissue comprised largely of ciliary processes of about 70 mg wet weight. Retina was teased gently from the posterior segment after removal of the vitreous, leaving most of the pigment epithelium *in situ*. Tissues were immersed in ice-cold 0·3 M mannitol until required.

Tissues were incubated in 10 ml Warburg flasks in a phosphate buffer (Riley, 1964a) or Krebs-Ringer bicarbonate (Umbreit, Burris and Stauffer, 1957), with the addition of 3·3 mM glucose. Sodium ions were replaced in the medium by Tris or choline, or ouabain was used at a concentration of 2×10^{-4} M, a level which had previously been shown to give complete inhibition of the Na-K ATPase of ciliary body (Riley, 1964b). The final volume, containing a half retina or whole ciliary strip, was 1·5 ml and the gas phase was 100% O_2; 100% N_2; 95% O_2/5% CO_2 or 95% N_2/5% CO_2. Temperature of incubation was 37° and was of 50 min duration for ciliary body and 40 min for retina. Glucose was measured by the glucose oxidase method (Marks, 1959) and lactate by the method of Barker and Summerson (1941).

3. Results

The inhibition of the Na-K ATPase by ouabain produced identical effects on the parameters measured to those observed when sodium ions were absent from the medium. Therefore in the results presented below no distinction has been made between the methods of inhibition.

Figures 1–4 show the effect of inhibition of sodium transport on the aerobic and anaerobic metabolism of ciliary body and retina. The most pronounced effect was upon the oxygen uptake and aerobic conversion of glucose to lactate by ciliary body. Under anaerobic conditions glycolysis of this tissue was not so severely affected. Quantitative differences were apparent in the degree of inhibition of retinal metabolism, under the different conditions studied, but in only one case did the inhibition not exceed 30%. This was the anaerobic glycolysis in phosphate buffer, the inhibited values being only 10% lower than the control values (Fig. 4).

In Fig. 5 the effect of 2, 4-dinitrophenol on the aerobic and anaerobic metabolism of ciliary body can be seen. Oxygen uptake was stimulated greatly in the controls, and by an almost equivalent amount in the ouabain inhibited flasks. Conversion of glucose to lactate was increased in the controls, but more so in the ouabain flasks, indicating a partial relief of the inhibition by dinitrophenol. This was more clearly seen under anaerobic conditions when the effect of dinitrophenol on the controls was less than aerobically and the relief of ouabain inhibition was enhanced.

Under anaerobic conditions in both tissues the inhibition of sodium transport caused an approximately equal decline in glucose utilization and lactate production and therefore the lactate: glucose ratio remained constant between 1·8 and 1·9. However, under aerobic conditions in phosphate buffer the ratio fell, indicating utilization of glucose by a different pathway. Experiments with [1-¹⁴C] and [6-¹⁴C]glucose showed that in ciliary body there was little utilization of the hexose monophosphate

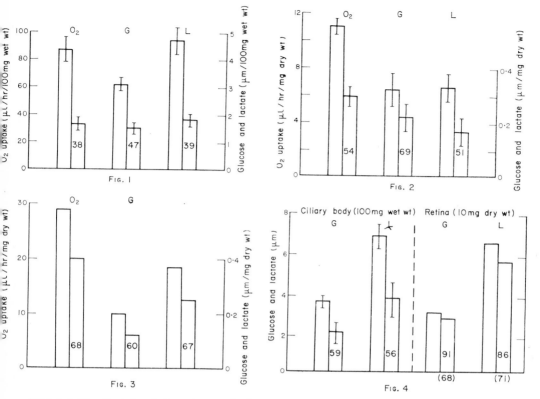

FIGS. 1–4. The effect of ouabain or absence of sodium ions on the glucose metabolism of ciliary body and retina. Figures in the right-hand columns indicate experimental activity expressed as % of control activity.

FIG. 1. Ciliary body in phosphate buffer and O_2.

FIG. 2. Retina in phosphate buffer and O_2.

FIG. 3. Retina in bicarbonate buffer and 95% O_2/5% CO_2.

FIG. 4. Anaerobic glycolysis in phosphate buffer and N_2. Figures in parentheses indicate % inhibition of retinal glycolysis in bicarbonate buffer.

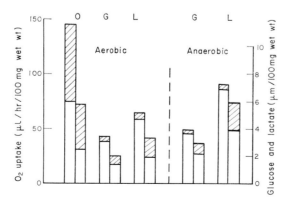

FIG. 5. The effect of 2, 4-dinitrophenol on control and ouabain-inhibited metabolism of ciliary body. Hatched areas represent the stimulation induced by DNP.

pathway under normal conditions (Table I). However, in the absence of sodium or when ouabain was present the fraction of glucose metabolized by this pathway was considerably increased. A single experiment with retina gave very similar results. The "specific activity" measurements were obtained by dividing the activity in cts/min

TABLE I

Effect of ouabain on production of $^{14}CO_2$ from [1-^{14}C] and [6-^{14}C]glucose by ciliary body

	Activity (cts/min)*		"Specific activity" (cts/min/$\mu l\ O_2$)	
	Control	Ouabain	Control	Ouabain
1-^{14}C	5950	1560	69	47
6-^{14}C	4690	580	54	18
Ratio C1/C6	1·3	2·7		

* Mean of 3 experiments.

by the oxygen uptake of the tissue, on the assumption that the respiratory quotient did not change appreciably in the presence of ouabain. It will be seen that the values with ouabain are lower than the controls, indicating that a greater proportion of the CO_2 has been produced from non-labelled substrates.

4. Discussion

It is clear from the above results that inhibition of sodium transport in ciliary body and retina leads to a marked decrease in the activity of both the respiratory and glycolytic systems. Inhibition of respiration under similar conditions has been found to occur in brain, liver and kidney, though in each case to a lesser extent than in the ocular tissues (Whittam and Blond, 1964; Elshove and van Rossum, 1963; Whittam and Willis, 1963), and recently, a small inhibition of glycolysis in erythrocytes has been shown (Whittam, Ager and Wiley, 1964). These results are explained by the regulatory effect of the Na-K ATPase on the ADP levels of the cell. When this enzyme is inhibited, either by ouabain or through lack of sodium ions, less ATP is hydrolysed, resulting in a lack of ADP which is essential for oxidative phosphorylation. Therefore, the electron transport system of the mitochondria is slowed down and oxygen uptake falls. Glycolysis also is ADP dependent and low levels of ADP will inhibit the 1, 3-diphosphoglycerate kinase and the phosphoenolpyruvate kinase steps. The effect of 2, 4-dinitrophenol which uncouples oxidative phosphorylation, but not the substrate level phosphorylations of glycolysis, and increases the Mg-ATPase of mitochondria, fits this hypothesis. The effect on respiration is clouded by the large stimulatory effect on the controls, but the relief of inhibition of glucose utilization and lactate formation probably results from increased levels of ADP in the soluble fraction of the cell. This is most apparent under anaerobic conditions where there is no complication due to stimulation of the tricarboxylic acid cycle.

Inhibition of 1, 3-diphosphoglycerate kinase will result in a lower rate of utilization of phosphorylated hexoses by the glycolytic system and consequently more glucose-6-phosphate will be available to glucose-6-phosphate dehydrogenase, the first enzyme of the hexose monophosphate pathway. Therefore, in the presence of ouabain, a relative increase in the proportion of glucose metabolized by this route is to be expected. It is of interest that in ciliary body and retina this pathway is apparently little utilized under normal conditions. Possibly this is because the route is largely used for synthetic purposes and is an inefficient route for energy production. Futterman (1963) has shown that NADPH produced by this pathway is used for the reduction of vitamin A aldehyde in the retina, but this is likely to contribute appreciably to total retinal glucose metabolism only *in vivo* or under specially designed *in vitro* conditions.

The lower specific activity of $^{14}CO_2$ found in the presence of ouabain indicates that endogenous substrates are being metabolized to a relatively greater extent than in the controls. This may be because ouabain-induced changes in the cell dynamics may favour the use of endogenous substrates, or more probably because the availability of exogenous glucose is decreased. In several tissues it has been shown that glucose uptake is a sodium dependent, ouabain-sensitive process (Csáky 1963; Schultz and Zalusky 1964) and it seems probable that as a result of decreased sodium transport across the ciliary epithelium the transport of glucose into the cells is also inhibited.

The results obtained in the present experiments do not permit conclusions to be drawn concerning the specific role that a high rate of aerobic glycolysis may play in ciliary or retinal metabolism. Both the secretion of aqueous humour and retinal function are oxygen dependent systems and, unlike the case of erythrocytes, glycolysis alone cannot support integrated function. The remarkable degree of cell specialization in the retina and the discrete localization of certain enzymes (especially the high lactic dehydrogenase activity of Müller fibres shown by Dr. Kuwabara in this Symposium) provide several possibilities for a specific role of glycolysis, although at which point it is impossible yet to determine. In the ciliary body the localization of the major part of the Na-K ATPase in the inner layer of cells, alongside the greater fraction of the respiratory activity (Cole, 1963, 1964), suggests that glycolysis may not participate in sodium extrusion *per se*. One possible role is in facilitating the passage of sodium from the blood through the outer layer of cells, making a constant supply available to the pump situated in the inner layer. Alternatively, a high rate of formation of lactate might be designed so that this anion could follow the extruded sodium out of the epithelial cells along with bicarbonate and chloride. There is a very high lactate content in the posterior chamber, probably more than can be accounted for by lens metabolism, and Cole (1963) showed that lactic dehydrogenase activity was present in both cell layers of the ciliary epithelium. These two postulates are not mutually exclusive and the glycolytic activity, which accounts for about 80% of the glucose utilization of ciliary body, may have other functions in addition to these.

REFERENCES

Barker, S. B. and Summerson, W. H. (1941). *J. biol. Chem.* **138**, 535.
Bonting, S. L., Simon, K. A. and Hawkins, N. M. (1961). *Archs. Biochem. Biophys.* **95**, 416.
Cole, D. F. (1961). *Br. J. Ophthal.* **45**, 641.
Cole, D. F. (1963). *Exp. Eye Res.* **2**, 284.
Cole, D. F. (1964). *Exp. Eye Res.* **3**, 72.
Csáky, T. Z. (1963). *Biochim. biophys. Acta* **74**, 160.
Elshove, A. and van Rossum, G. D. V. (1963). *J. Physiol.* **168**, 531.
Futterman, S. (1963). *J. biol. Chem.* **238**, 1145.
Marks, V. (1959). *Clin. chim. Acta* **4**, 395.
Riley, M. V. (1964a). *Nature, Lond.* (In press)
Riley, M. V. (1964b). *Exp. Eye Res.* **3**, 76.
Schultz, S. G. and Zalusky, R. (1964). *J. gen. Physiol.* **47**, 1043.
Skou, J. C. (1960). *Biochim. biophys. Acta* **42**, 6.

Umbreit, W. W., Burris, R. H. and Stauffer, J. F. (1957). *Manometric Techniques*. Burgess
    Publishing Co., Minneapolis.
Whittam, R. and Blond, D. M. (1964). *Biochem. J.* **92**, 147.
Whittam, R. and Willis, J. S. (1963). *J. Physiol.* **168**, 158.
Whittam, R., Ager, M. E. and Wiley, J. S. (1964). *Nature, Lond.* **202**, 1111.

DISCUSSION

Dr. Reading felt that, in view of the close similarity between the retina and the ciliary body, was it not possible that the high glucose utilization and glycolytic activity of the ciliary body was involved in the production of glutamate rather than the provision of lactate as a carrier anion for potassium. He was referring to the direct production of glutamate from glucose as reported for brain tissue.

Dr. Riley explained that although there was evidence of glutamate production in the ciliary body—indeed glutamate and aspartate were the principal amino acids produced from glucose—nevertheless, glutamate production did not seem to be as high as in the retina. A further distinction lay in the failure of the ciliary body to produce gamma amino butyric acid.

Dr. Reading thought that, in view of Krebs' work showing the importance of glutamate in maintaining the potassium content of the retina, it might well have special significance in a secretory tissue such as the ciliary body.

Dr. Cole described his own experiences, prompted by the work of Krebs, in which he had found some effect of glutamate on the K content of the ciliary body, but that further experiments failed to reveal any dramatic effect on the transport mechanism as a whole.

Dr. Pedler stressed the similarity, from the standpoint of electron microscopic studies, between the non-pigmented outer layers of the ciliary body and the radial fibres of the retina. In view of the computer-like complexity of the latter, however, he felt this was sufficient justification for an augmented energy system.

Dr. Ames said that he and his colleagues had been most interested in Krebs' findings and had attempted to repeat some of his work. The conditions were somewhat different, Krebs employed retinas that had been removed in ice-water, and the ion exchange had thus been enhanced. Glutamate, under these conditions, induced a considerable uptake of potassium, although it was not clear whether this was accompanied by water and whether, therefore, the actual concentration of potassium was changed.

In his own experiments, he had minimized post-mortem changes and observed two effects. First, sodium, potassium and water were accumulated in the first hour, and if one assumed that glutamate was the equivalent ion, the water uptake was sufficient to render the tissue isotonic. Under this hypothesis, i.e., that glutamate was equivalent in this respect to the total sodium and potassium, the calculated glutamate uptake was as found by Krebs. Dr. Ames pointed out that although this appeared a reasonable phenomenon, further studies showed that in the first 10 min there was a loss of potassium and a gain of sodium. It appeared that during the whole hour there was a total gain of sodium plus potassium, but that the individual ions varied. In answer to a query from Dr. Futterman regarding the level of ouabain used, Dr. Riley agreed that he had approached the problems by using a large level (10^{-4} M) which would induce 100% inhibition of the Na/K ATP-ase of the tissue. Direct effects of ouabain on glycolytic or respiratory enzymes had not been reported.

Dr. Futterman suggested that it would be of value to add hexokinase to the system in order to provide a plentiful supply of ADP. Dr. Riley agreed that further experiments were required before any firm concept regarding the mode of action of ouabain could be established, but pointed out that absence of sodium produced an identical picture.

Selective Action of Chemical Agents on Individual Retinal Layers*

ALBERT M. POTTS

The Eye Research Laboratories, University of Chicago, Chicago, Illinois, U.S.A.

The structure of the retina—comprising layers of functionally different cells in extremely close juxtaposition—has embarrassed biochemists for half a century. The inability to attribute a particular biochemical or physiological response to a particular functional cell group has severely hampered progress in retinal physiology.

In recent times the microdissections of Lowry have contributed significantly to biochemical knowledge, but the technique requires destruction of retinal organization. An alternative approach is the use of substances which selectively destroy individual retinal layers. This attack has several virtues. (1) It leaves the remainder of the retina accessible for physiological study. (2) Investigation of the mechanism of selective damage gives valuable information on the individuality of the cell layer in question. (3) The combination of several agents makes it theoretically possible to produce retinas with a single cell population *in situ*.

Perhaps because the normal retinal cleavage separates the pigment epithelium from the rest of the retina, this layer has received little attention. Knowledge that the resting potential of the eye and, indeed, vision itself, depend on the integrity of this layer has stimulated work in a number of laboratories. Iodate, azide and diaminodiphenoxyalkanes all cause damage to pigment epithelium.

Iodoacetate has been used by several groups to destroy the receptor cell layer and metabolic studies have been made on retinas before and after treatment. Dithizone was erroneously thought to have a similarly selective effect on the retinal receptors. Oxygen and fluoride are effective to some extent.

The bipolar cell layer of mice was found to be destroyed by large doses of glutamate and formation of the ganglion cell layer was prevented. Investigation of the electrophysiology of the remaining retina and of the mechanism of glutamate action has been further explored.

Selective destruction of the ganglion cell layer can be obtained by retrograde degeneration after optic nerve section. Only recently has information become available that selective destruction of ganglion cells can be achieved chemically by N-nitroso-β-chlorethylcarbamate.

The possibilities for fruitful investigation along the three directions outlined above have by no means been exhausted. A number of new lines of investigation can be detailed and it is anticipated that much new information on retinal function will be derived from selectively retinotoxic substances.

1. Introduction

One of the greatest hindrances to the study of retinal function lies in the anatomy of the retina. The closely adherent multi-layered structure in which each layer must have its own individual physiological function and metabolic activity is the base of the problem. Studies of "whole retina", that is, retina minus the pigment epithelial layer, can only represent a very gross kind of average. One type of solution to this problem is that obtained by Lowry who separated extremely minute quantities of each of the retinal layers by microdissection of frozen, dried, retinal sections and then performed microchemical enzymatic studies on this material (Lowry, 1956). An alternative approach, which in the opinion of this writer has not yet been fully exploited, offers real promise in understanding of differences between individual retinal layers. This is the study of the effect of toxic substances which specifically affect only a single retinal layer coupled with the study of retinal function after the action

* Supported in part by United States Public Health Service grants no. NB–02522 and NB–02523.

of such substances or combinations of substances. The study of the mechanism of the toxic effect on an individual retinal layer gives specific information on the individuality of the layer; study of the retina minus that particular layer compared to studies on retinas with that particular intact give information on the normal metabolism of the substructure in question. A considerable amount of energy has been expended in search for such specifically acting substances and some studies have been made on the mechanism of toxicity. However, much remains to be done. It is with a discussion of what has been accomplished and what remains to be accomplished in this area that the rest of this essay will be concerned.

2. Pigment Epithelium

To set some arbitrary pattern, the treatment will be of individual layers from the most exterior to the most interior. It happens that the most exterior layer, the pigment epithelium, was the earliest one found to be destroyed by a specific toxic agent. In the pre-antibiotic era of the 1920's attempts were made to combat systemic septic disease, such as septicemia, by intravenous injection of inorganic antiseptics. It was found after the use of one of these—concentrated Pregl solution, known under the trade name of Septojod—that a number of individuals became blind (Riehm, 1927). It was demonstrated by Riehm (1929) that the primary retinal involvement was of the pigment epithelium and that this disease could be induced experimentally by injecting Septojod into pigmented rabbits. In 1935, Vito (1935) was able to demonstrate that the actual toxic agent involved was sodium iodate. However, the exact way in which iodate causes degeneration and the reason for the particular susceptibility of the pigment epithelium has not been adequately worked out. Although iodate is known for its property as a relatively stable oxidizing agent, and though the probability of this mechanism of action is reinforced by the fact that the iodate effect can be completely neutralized by the reducing agent, cysteine (Sorsby and Harding, 1960a), the effect has not been reproduced by other oxidizing agents, such as manganese dioxide, perborate and persulfate (Sorsby, 1941). It is true, however, that none of these agents has the relative stability of iodate, and a dose comparable to that of iodate could not be given intravenously without killing the experimental animals. Thus, much remains to be done with this remarkable and highly specific reaction.

A second series of drugs which apparently selectively affect the pigment epithelium is the set of diaminodiphenoxyalkanes (Edge, Mason, Wien and Ashton, 1956). In susceptible animals; monkey, dog and cat, a single oral or intravenous dose causes eventual pigmented retinopathy and (Nakajima, 1958) complete loss of the electroretinogram within a period of several days. These effects are apparently also due to selective action on the retinal pigment epithelium. However, since receptor cell outer segments are apparently not viable in the absence of functioning pigment epithelium, secondary degeneration of receptor cells occurs consistently; and one is no longer dealing with loss of a single retinal layer.

An alternative method for studying pigment epithelium metabolism is a mechanical one, since after removal of the rest of the retina at its normal cleavage site, careful brushing of the residual optic cup allows preparation of pigment epithelium in uncontaminated condition; and *in vitro* studies of this cell suspension can be made (Glocklin and Potts, 1962). Studies of the normal functioning of such pigment epithelium suspensions and the effect on these functions of the known toxic substances are being conducted by Dr. Vera Glocklin. Inhibition of the uptake of phosphorus into the acid-soluble organic fraction of pigment epithelium has been reported by her (Glocklin and Potts, 1962).

3. Receptor Cells

A great deal of attention has been paid to agents which cause degeneration of the retinal receptors, particularly the rods. The most dramatic and thorough of these phenomena is the destruction of rod cells by carefully controlled doses of iodoacetate, given intravenously in rabbits (Schubert and Bornschein, 1951; Noell, 1952). Production of the effect in rats with the aid of sodium malate was demonstrated by Graymore and Tansley (1959a).

Here, too, despite the large amount of work that has been done in the area, the mechanism is still not completely established. As is well known, iodoacetate is a classical inhibitor of glycolysis and works by means of its properties as a sulfhydryl reagent. It is true that cysteine is highly effective in preventing retinal degeneration after iodoacetate (Sorsby and Harding, 1960a). It is further true that Graymore and Tansley (1959b) have demonstrated severe inhibition of glycolysis in the rat retina immediately after injection of a dose which will eventually cause visual cell degeneration. However, with other known sulfhydryl inhibitors, such as iodoacetamide, 1-fluoro-2, 6-dinitrobenzene, or sodium parachloromercuribenzoate, no such degeneration could be produced (Sorsby, Newhouse and Lucas, 1957). It should be noted here again, that systemic toxicity of the other more effective thiol reagents prevented attaining a systemic dose equal in molarity to that of the iodoacetate and could be responsible for the lack of effect.

A tempting alternative hypothesis for the mechanism of iodoacetate action is based on the demonstration by Wald and Brown (1951–52) that free-sulfhydryl groups in opsin are required for synthesis of rhodopsin from retinene. Reaction with these and disorganization of the outer segment might be the key to toxic activity. However, in *in vitro* experiments the synthesis of rhodopsin is not affected by iodoacetate and is blocked by very dilute solutions of parachloromercuribenzoate. Thus, it is hard to attribute visual cell degeneration to this mechanism. Furthermore, the electron microscope studies of Lasansky and De Robertis (1959) show simultaneous degeneration of the outer segments, the inner segments and the synaptic layer after treatment by iodoacetate. Thus, despite the objections noted above, inhibition of glycolysis by a relatively nontoxic agent seems to be the best way to explain destruction of receptor cells by iodoacetate.

Studies on retinas deprived of their visual cells by iodoacetate treatment and allowed to recover from the acute effects of iodoacetate poisoning show marked, long-term, decrease of glycolytic activity, suggesting strongly that the receptor cells account for a significant proportion of the glycolysis of whole retina (Graymore and Tansley, 1959b; Noell, 1955). However, these two observations represent the only chemical work done to date on retinas minus receptor cells.

To further complicate the picture there are apparently other toxic substances which may cause extensive visual cell destruction and presumably by different mechanisms. First, pure oxygen at atmospheric pressure for 48 hr can cause loss of more than 60% of the retinal receptors in an adult rabbit. Oxygen at 1·6 atm. can cause complete cell destruction (Noell, 1958). Curiously, both iodoacetate and oxygen are ineffective in young animals below 20 days of age. No adequate mechanism has been advanced to explain this phenomenon. A second substance which causes destruction of visual cells together with some pigment epithelium is fluoride (Sorsby and Harding, 1960b). At levels which cause the retinal effect, 15–20% of the animals are killed and only another 15 or 20% show the effect. The known inhibitory action of fluoride on enolase, an indispensable enzyme in glycolysis, may well be at the basis of this effect. The fact that fluoride must act by complexing magnesium, vital to the reaction, and must therefore be present in relatively high concentrations probably accounts for both the toxicity and the low rate of affected animals.

Although dithizone (diphenylthiocarbazone) was originally reported to cause visual cell destruction similar to that caused by iodoacetate (Butturini, Grignolo and Baronchelli, 1953), later studies suggest that all retinal layers are affected by this chelating agent for heavy metals. Late optic atrophy, secondary to ganglion cell degeneration, is a constant feature of dithizone poisoning (Quaranta and Bozza, 1959). Thus, although interesting in its own right, this substance should not be considered in the same category as those which selectively affect receptor cells nor need the mechanism of toxic action be identical.

4. Bipolar Cells

An entirely different type of selective destruction of retinal elements is that observed following the administration of sodium glutamate in relatively high doses to newborn rats and mice. This effect, first reported by Lucas and Newhouse (1957), is not easily obtained in adult animals in contrast to the iodoacetate and oxygen effects mentioned above. In animals treated with glutamate the ganglion cell layer degenerates and the inner nuclear layer fails to differentiate, leaving a practically pure culture of receptor cells in an animal allowed to develop to 3 months of age. Such animals show a characteristic loss of the b-wave with preservation only of the a-wave in the electroretinogram (Potts, Modrell and Kingsbury, 1960). Submaximal treatment was characterized by temporary abolition of the b-wave and its later restoration along with growth of the bipolar cell layer. Even in optimally treated animals there is a ragged layer of cells, usually two cells thick, which persists at 3 months of age and which are perhaps responsible for the relatively rapid return of the negative a-wave to the base line rather than producing a more extended negative response.

Even more interesting is the effect of changing the intensity of the light stimulus to the eyes of animals well treated with sodium glutamate (but still possessing the bipolar cell residue). Stimuli of threshold intensity and a bit greater, produced only a cornea-positive b-wave-like response of low amplitude. To these positive responses were added the negative, shorter latency, a-wave at higher intensities. At still higher intensities, only the large a-wave was recordable for it swamped out any residual positivity (Plate 1) (Potts and Buckser, unpublished results).

If treated animals are allowed to survive for an additional 3-month-period, this last layer of bipolar cells appears to degenerate. At this time there is some additional loss of receptor cells as well. The electroretinographic response is a smaller than normal electronegative wave of sustained negativity (Potts and Buckser, 1964). Staining the normal rat retina with cresyl violet for Nissl substance showed complete absence of such material near the nuclei of the receptor cells and the presence of Nissl material near virtually every nucleus in the bipolar and ganglion cell layers (Plate 2). In an animal 6 months after treatment with sodium glutamate there was no trace of Nissl substance in the layer of nuclei, apparently receptor cell nuclei (Plate 3).

In the case of the glutamate effect it was possible to study more intensively the mechanism of action, and on the strong possibility that one might be dealing with enzyme repression, a series of enzyme activities were determined in the retinas of normal and treated animals (Freedman and Potts, 1962). Figure 1 shows the re-lationship between glutamine, glutamic acid and α-ketoglutarate, and the enzymes

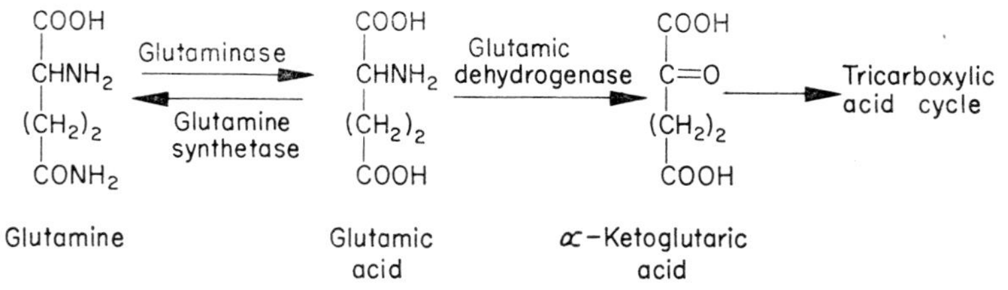

FIG. 1. Enzymatic relations of glutamic acid.

that are responsible for these interchanges. In addition glutamotransferase (not shown on the figure) is able to catalyze the transfer of glutamyl radical from glutamine to other amine receptors. If, as we postulated, the presence of large quantities of glutamic acid tend to repress enzymes that would form glutamic acid from glutamine, then glutaminase levels in treated retinas should be lower than in normal controls. This was found to be the case. Furthermore, the presence of glutamic acid might well induce the increased synthesis of enzymes which would be able to remove it from the reaction site. Such an enzyme is glutamic-oxalacetic transaminase and, in fact, the concentration of this enzyme was found to be increased (Freedman and Potts, 1963).

It was suggested by Waelsch (1955) that the set of glutamate enzyme systems might be responsible for controlling the amount of α-ketoglutarate available to the cell, and consequently the rate of tricarboxylic acid cycle operation. With the enzyme changes accomplished by glutamate treatment, the retinas of treated animals should have an excess of glutamine and a deficit of glutamic acid caused by deficit of glu-taminase and excess of transaminase. This situation would paralyze the control of the tricarboxylic acid cycle as postulated. Another alternative is that the high con-centration of glutamate and the increased amount of transaminase might result in net liberation within the cell, or within the region, of large amounts of ammonia and consequent toxicity.

Additional studies threw some light on the reason why the effect was restricted to newborn animals. The uptake of glutamate in rat retina which was found to be quite large in 5-day-old animals dropped sharply with age to a quarter or less of its previous values (Freedman and Potts, 1963). Thus the establishment of a retinal barrier against glutamate well on its way by the 10th day would be reason enough that subsequent injection would have little effect on the retinas of the animal studied.

An hitherto unpublished set of experiments concern themselves with the localiza-tion of glutaminase in the tissue of the rat. This was accomplished by the set of reactions, shown in Fig. 2. (α-Naphthyl glutamine was synthesized by a commercial house and the fast blue salt was the gift of the National Aniline Corp.) On hydrolysis of the naphthyl glutamine the liberated naphthylamine coupled with the fast blue B salt and gave rise to locally deposited dye. Our retinas were incubated at 37°C and pH 7·4 for 2 hr. During this time rod outer segments were lost, but the rest of the retina was preserved intact. The retinas were embedded in gelatin and sectioned while the gelatin block was frozen. Some of the thawed sections were counterstained with malachite green to contrast with the orange-red color produced by the dye reaction. Others were observed unstained. Surprisingly, the highest concentration of

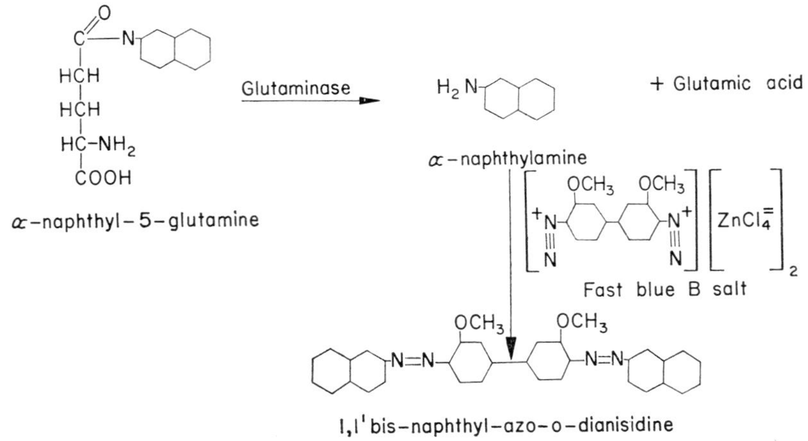

FIG. 2. Histochemical reaction for glutaminase.

glutaminase was found in the inner and outer reticular layers rather than in the layer of bipolar cell nuclei. Nevertheless, it is conceivable that enzymatic activity here could have definite effect on the bipolar cells (Plate 4). Thus, we have come to know considerably more about the toxic reaction of glutamate with the retina than was known at one time. The resulting preparation and essentially pure culture of receptor cells has not yet been adequately exploited for metabolic studies and such studies are now under way in our laboratory.

5. Ganglion Cell Layer

It would not be proper to conclude this discussion of effect of chemicals on individual retinal layers without mentioning the one substance known to selectively affect the ganglion cell layer of the retina. In an NDRC report now declassified, Gates and Renshaw (1946) described the extensive chromatolysis and destruction of retinal ganglion cells in the eyes of cats allowed to inhale a concentration of 50 $\mu g/l$ for 10 min of the vapor of methyl-N-β-chlorethyl-N-nitrosocarbamate.

$$Cl—CH_2—CH_2—N—C—OCH_3$$
$$\underset{NO}{|} \quad \underset{O}{\diagdown}$$

It was reported by the same workers that nitrogen mustard did not give this type of ganglion cell destruction. The nitrosocarbamate which behaves chemically in a manner similar to nitrogen mustard is able to destroy oxygen uptake in tissues *in vitro* at M/1000, leaving glycolysis intact. Here, then, we may be dealing with a mechanism of specific destruction of a single cell layer based not on interference with glycolysis but on interference with an oxidative process. Because of the vesicant nature of the substance in question and general difficulty in handling it, its use as an

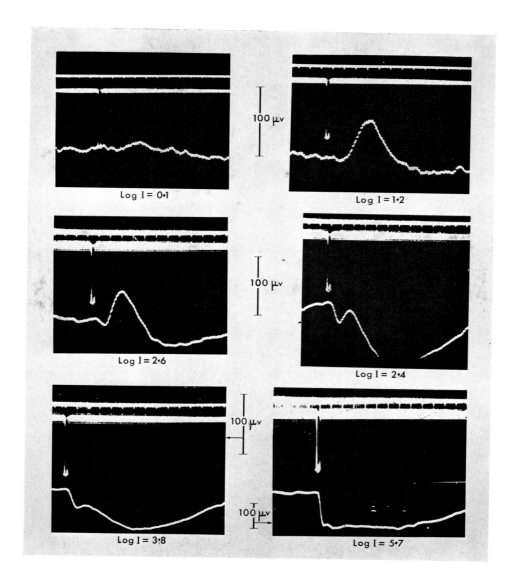

PLATE 1. The effect of increasing light intensity on the electro-retinogram of the glutamate-treated rat (time mark = 50 msec).

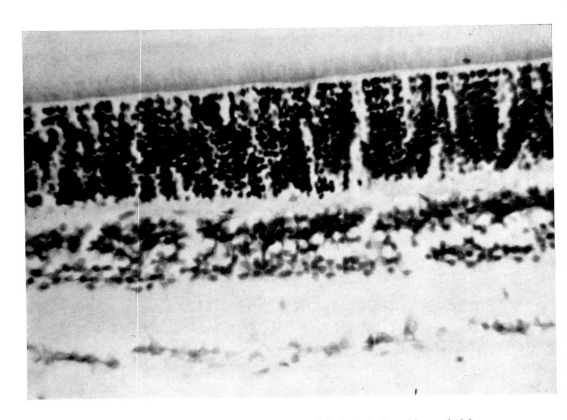

PLATE 2. Normal rat retina (6 months) stained for Nissl bodies with cresyl violet.

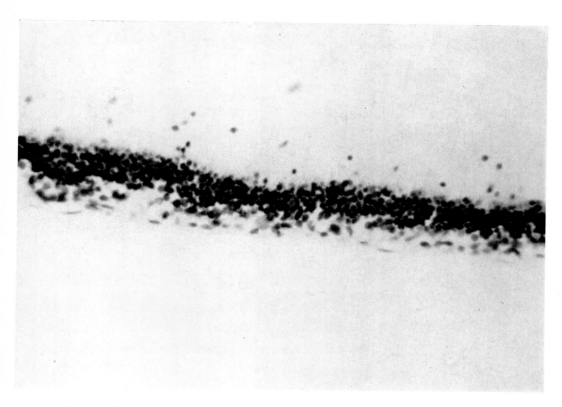

PLATE 3. Glutamate-treated rat retina (6 months) stained for Nissl bodies with cresyl violet.

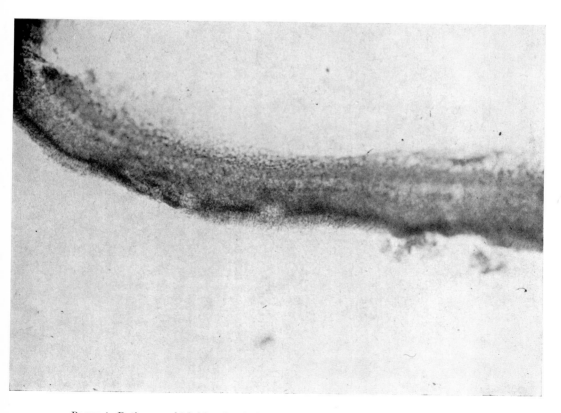

PLATE 4. Retina on which histochemical reaction for glutaminase has been carried out.

agent to eliminate the ganglion cells will probably not become popular. The same effect can be achieved with perhaps greater ease and sureness by intracranial section of the optic nerve. However, study of the mechanism of action of the nitrosocarbamate should again lead to specific knowledge about the cell layer in question.

Although much study remains to be done, it is hoped that this discussion has pointed out the virtues of the investigation of agents which can selectively destroy individual retinal layers. Such investigation leads to greater knowledge of the metabolism and the unique features of the physiology of the particular retinal layer and the result, a preparation now lacking the retinal layer in question, is in itself a subject for physiological examination.

REFERENCES

Butturini, U., Grignolo, A. and Baronchelli, A. (1953). *G. clin. Med.* **34**, 1253.
Edge, N. D., Mason, D. F., Wien, R. and Ashton, N. (1956). *Nature, Lond.* **178**, 806.
Freedman, J. K. and Potts, A. M. (1962). *Invest. Ophthal.* **1**, 118.
Freedman, J. K. and Potts, A. M. (1963). *Invest. Ophthal.* **2**, 252.
Gates, M. and Renshaw, B. (1946). Chemical Warfare Agents and Related Chemical Problems. Sum. Tech. Rept. Div. 9 NDRC, Washington.
Glocklin, V. C. and Potts, A. M. (1962). *Invest. Ophthal.* **1**, 111.
Graymore, C. N. and Tansley, K. (1959a). *Br. J. Ophthal.* **43**, 177.
Graymore, C. N. and Tansley, K. (1959b). *Br. J. Ophthal.* **43**, 486.
Lasansky, A. and De Robertis, E. (1959). *J. biophys. biochem. Cytol.* **5**, 245.
Lowry, O. H., Roberts, N. R. and Lewis, C. (1956). *J. biol. Chem.* **220**, 879.
Lucas, D. R. and Newhouse, J. P. (1957). *Arch. Ophthal.* **58**, 193.
Nakajima, A. (1958). *Ophthalmologica, Basel* **136**, 332.
Noell, W. K. (1952). *J. cell. comp. Physiol.* **40**, 25.
Noell, W. K. (1955). *Am. J. Ophthal.* **40**, 60.
Noell, W. K. (1958). *Arch. Ophthal.* **60**, 702.
Potts, A. M., Modrell, R. W. and Kingsbury, C. (1960). *Am. J. Ophthal.* **50**, 900.
Quaranta, C. A. and Vozza, R. (1959). *Boll. Oculist.* **38**, 665.
Riehm, W. (1927). *Klin. Mbl. Augenheilk.* **78**, 87.
Riehm, W. (1929). *Arch. Augenheilk.* **100/101**, 872.
Schubert, G. and Bornschein, H. (1951). *Experientia* **7**, 461.
Sorsby, A. (1941). *Br. J. Ophthal.* **25**, 62.
Sorsby, A. and Harding, R. (1960a). *Nature, Lond.* **187**, 608.
Sorsby, A. and Harding, R. (1960b). *Br. J. Ophthal.* **44**, 213.
Sorsby, A., Newhouse, J. P. and Lucas, D. R. (1957). *Br. J. Ophthal.* **41**, 309.
Vito, P. (1935). *Boll. Oculist.* **14**, 945.
Waelsch, H. (1955). In *Neurochemistry*, p. 173, ed. by K. A. C. Elliott, I. H. Page and J. H. Quastel. Thomas, Springfield.
Wald, G. and Brown, P. K. (1951–52). *J. gen. Physiol.* **35**, 797.

DISCUSSION

DR. READING stressed that the variety of effects induced by different chemical inhibitors reflected the intricacy of the tissue itself. He was particularly interested in the role of sulphydryl groups. Dr. Reading had recently applied amperometric titration methods to the estimation of free and acid soluble SH groups in the rabbit retina, a method depending on the saturation of the tissue with para-chloromercuribenzoate and subsequent back titration with cysteine. He found that after iodate and diaminodiphenoxyalkane the value at first fluctuates, but rises thereafter. On the other hand, after iodoacetate the total remains the same, but the acid soluble sulphydryl fraction falls abruptly. Dr. Reading took these preliminary findings to suggest that the first two reagents caused considerable denaturation, and certainly endorsed the view that many of these compounds acted in entirely different ways. As regards glutamate, he thought that the recent work of Richter was relevant in which he had demonstrated that in the brain the carbon skeleton of glucose was converted into glutamate before entering into oxidation. He thought that this might apply in the inner layers of the retina and if so, would be of importance in interpreting the phenomenon described.

PROFESSOR BONAVITA referred to a more recent publication by Krebs contradicting Richter's conclusions. DR. READING agreed with the fact that there was some doubt about this glutamate formation, and in reply to a question from Professor Cohen explained that the pathway suggested by Richter did not involve the Krebs cycle.

PROFESSOR COHEN also discussed the intricacies and importance of metabolic control by repression or induction of specific enzymes, although he stressed the difficulties of defining the extent of influence of such reactions. He quoted, as an example, the work of Dr. Sanwal from Manitoba, who had demonstrated two glutamic dehydrogenases in neurospora. One, required for synthesis of glutamate, required NADP as the coenzyme, whereas the degradative counterpart was NAD dependent. Glutamate concentration affected these two reactions in opposite directions, and one could imagine that such a situation might have far reaching effects as a regulatory mechanism.

DR. AMES raised the interesting point that on the basis of work he had done, was it not possible that high concentrations of glutamate might exert an osmotic physical action, rather than an enzymatic functional one. He suggested that it might be of use to try the effects of the α-isomer to discriminate between these phenomena. Although DR. POTTS felt that the confinement of the effect to the immature animal was indicative of a physiogical function, DR. AMES reminded him that this was a permeability phenomenom.

DR. KUWABARA described some electron microscope findings of his laboratory on iodoacetate treated rats. He found that the early changes, occuring within a few hours, were centred on the synaptic region, and that the outer segments remained normal until about 24 hr. PROFESSOR POTTS replied that he had quoted the work of Lasansky and De Robertis to demonstrate that the primary lesion was not exclusive to the outer segment. Dr. Kuwabara's evidence was an even more convincing argument against the involvement in the damage of any mechanism involving rhodopsin synthesis.

DR. PEDLER, referring to these findings, suggested that the results of Lasansky and De Robertis were based on the use of methacrylate as an embedding agent, and were open to doubt, but PROFESSOR POTTS pointed out that no such changes were apparent in the control sections.

PROFESSOR NOELL stressed that it was important when interpreting data to remember that considerable species differences affected both the anatomical and electrophysiological effects of iodoacetate.

DR. ARDEN referred to one of Professor Potts' slides of a retina taken from a glutamate animal in which total destruction of the retina seemed to have occurred. He asked whether this was the normal end result if the retina was allowed to survive for sufficiently long following treatment. PROFESSOR POTTS explained that this was an isolated case, 6 months after treatment. He did not know whether this was the invariable result but thought it should be investigated.

DR. ARDEN added that he was disturbed by the long b-wave that Professor Potts obtained from animals almost lacking bipolar cells. Ischaemia of the retinal circulation, for example, led to a pure P.III. PROFESSOR POTTS, in reply, explained that a single high intensity did lead to a P.III, but DR. ARDEN said his results were the reverse of this, namely that the b-wave was only obtained at high intensity, presumably because greater intensity of stimulus was necessary for the elicitation of a response from the residual bipolars. PROFESSOR POTTS agreed this was a problem to consider further, and in reply to a comment from PROFESSOR COHEN agreed that this might not be a true b-wave, but a response from the receptor cells. This he had considered.

Notified Contribution to Discussion
More Thoughts on Ubiquinones

T. F. SLATER

*Department of Pathology, University College Hospital Medical School,
London, England*

I would like to make a few speculations concerning the results given in several of the papers presented to this Symposium. The major point concerns what is for me a very interesting finding, reported by Dr. Pearse, that ubiquinone or substances very closely related to ubiquinone are concentrated in the outer segments of the retina. One wonders what the function of this metabolically very active material is to justify this rather limited localization. One possibility could be connected with the known inhibitory action of vitamin E-like compounds—to which the ubiquinones bear a close relationship—on lipid peroxidation.

Lipid rich structures can be very susceptible to peroxidative reactions which occur in many tissues under certain conditions and cause very pronounced damage to structure and associated function. Lipid peroxidation reactions have recently been studied by Ernster and colleagues (CIBA Symposium *"Cellular Injury"*, 1964) in rat liver and rat brain microsomal preparations which contain lipid rich membranes presumably of a similar nature to those in the retinal outer segments. Lipid peroxidation as an example of free radical chain formation must be a nasty process as far as cellular organization is concerned.

In rat liver (and brain) microsomes, lipid peroxidation can be coupled to $NADPH_2$ oxidation *via* a flavoprotein, possibly the same as in $NADPH_2$-cytochrome *c* reductase (Hochstein and Ernster, 1963). Ascorbate, also, can be coupled to lipid peroxidation in microsomal fractions and one suggested scheme (Hochstein and Ernster, 1963) is

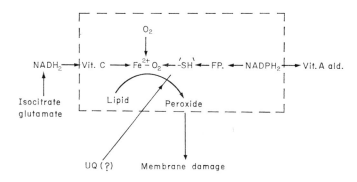

shown in the diagram within the dotted rectangle. It can be seen that the peroxidative reaction is suggested to proceed *via* a ferrous ion-oxygen complex; evidence has been reported that ADP is also necessary at this stage. FP and "–SH" stand for flavoprotein and a requirement for reduced sulphydryl-groups, respectively (Hochstein and Ernster, 1963).

L *

Dr. Heath has demonstrated that microsomal preparations from retinae will catalyse the oxidation of $NADH_2$ *via* ascorbate to cytochrome b_5. It seems possible that such microsomal fractions contain at least some fragmented remains of the lipid layers of the outer membranes. Thus, part of the vitamin C-cytochrome b_5 reductase activity could be present in the outer segments and could conceivably proceed along the route shown in the diagram with cytochrome b_5 perhaps accepting somewhere in the flavoprotein region. If so, then a system potentially capable of lipid peroxidation would be present. The $NADH_2$ necessary to prime the vitamin C reaction described by Dr. Heath could be provided by isocitric or glutamic dehydrogenases reported present in the outer segments by Dr. Pearse.

The speculation I wish to make is this. In such an orientated array as the outer segments (subjected to light radiation which might also favour radical formation) any sort of peroxidative reactions would be very deleterious. Is then the function of the 'ubiquinone' partly that of a protector against lipid peroxidation which would seem to me to be an important necessary requirement for such a system in which an active vitamin C-oxidizing system could be present? The peroxidation of lipid by such a system in rat liver has been shown to be inhibited by a vitamin E derivative (Hochstein and Ernster, 1963).

Thus, in the normal retina the high ubiquinone level might be necessary to prevent peroxidation in the presence of an active hydrogen transfer route through ascorbate and flavoprotein. If this is functional in the outer segments it could result in the reduction of NADP, thus providing a supply of $NADPH_2$ for alcohol dehydrogenase and the reduction of vitamin A aldehyde (see Futterman, this Symposium).

In animals or patients with a greatly decreased level of ubiquinone (or even a normal level but a disturbed spatial orientation) presumably the lipid peroxidation route could open up and damage to the lipid membranes would result. A peroxidative reaction, by providing a source of free radicals, could also lead to lysosomal damage (Tappel, 1963)—an alternative route of lysosomal injury to the hypothesis proposed yesterday by Dr. Newhouse based on vitamin A induced effects. In this connection, Dr. Campbell reported that vitamin A was reduced in the plasma of retinitis rats but vitamin A levels in the retina under these conditions are apparently not known. Perhaps retinal lysosomes anyway are 'adapted' to their environment of high vitamin A in a way found for retinal mitochondria (Wang, Slater and Dartnall, 1963). In that work it was found that retinal mitochondria did not swell on addition of vitamin A unlike their counterparts from liver.

REFERENCES

CIBA Symposium (1964). *Cellular Injury*. Churchill, London.
Hochstein, P. and Ernster, L. (1963). *Biochem. Biophys. Res. Comm.* **12**, 288.
Tappel, A. L., Sawant, P. L. and Shibka, S. (1963). *Lysosomes*. CIBA Symposium. Churchill, London.
Wang, D. Y., Slater, T. F. and Dartnall, J. H. A. (1963). *Vision Res.* **3**, 171.

A

Akiya, H., 47
Ames, A., III *22–29*, 48, 49, 50, 97, 114, 127, 154, 162
Amore, G., 86
Andrews, J. S., 17, 19
Arden, G. B., 2, 13, 21, 29, 49, *91–92*, 162
Ashton, N., 115, 120, 121, 124, 136, 137, 138, 147, 148, 156

B

Babel, J., 58
Bannister, R., 120, 121
Bastenie, P. A., et al., 123
Beaconsfield, P., 81
Beck, T. C., 133
Becker, B., 137, 139
Berkow, J. W., 83
Blach, R., 120
Bliss, A. F., 16
Bloodworth, J. M. B., 137, 148
Bonavita, V., *5–13*, 86, 89, 91, 162
Bonting, S. L., 55
Bornschein, H., 157
Bourne, M. C., 53, 54, 74, 91
Bridges, C., 3, 21, 49
Brotherton, J., 10, 11, 75
Brown, H. A., *115–122*, 138
Brown, I. K., 124
Brown, K. T., 47, 49
Brown, P. K., 157
Brückner, R., 54
Buckser, 158
Butturini, U., et al., 158

C

Cameron, E., *99*
Campbell, D. A., 53, 74, 89, 91, 114, 164
Caravaggio, L. L., 55
Chlouverakis, C., *123–138*
Cogan, D. G., 55, 83, 93, 94, 107, 120, 124, 135, 140, 143
Cohen, L., 7, 11, 13, 21, 29, *36–50*, 59, 60, 61, 62, 64, 71, 83, 84, 85, 89, 97, 113, 162
Cole, D. F., 29, 49, 90, *99*, 149, 153, 154
Cook, C., 121
Crapper, D. R., 26, 57

D

Dartnall, J. H. A., 164
Davson, H., 71
De Robertis, E., 4, 55, 62, 74, 112, 157, 162

De Roetth, A., Jr., 15
DiPaolo, J. A., 54, 55
Dowling, J. E., 4, 10, 20, 53, 55, 56, 68, 74, 89, 91
Duncan, L. J. P., et al., 123
Dunlop, D. M., 124

E

Edge, N. D., et al., 156
Engelson, G., 124
Enoch, J., 113
Eranko, O., et al., 47
Esmann, V., et al., 124
Everson Pearse, see Pearse

F

Falk, G., 47
Farkas, T. G., *31–35*, 133
Fatt, P., 47
Fiddick, R., *14–15*
Field, R. A., 124
Fine, B. S., 93
Folkers, 114
Forgacs, J., 10
Foulds, W. S., 91
Freedman, J. K., 159
Futterman, S., 12, 13, *16–21*, 49, 81, 83, 86, 87, 93, 114, 122, 153, 154, 164

G

Gates, M., 160
Glocklin, V. C., 156, 157
Gray, C. H., 133
Graymore, C. N., 6, 10, 11, 12, 18, 38, 40, 44, 55, 60, 64, 75, *83–90*, *115–122*, 134, 138, 157
Gruneberg, H., 54
Guarneri, R., 7, 10, 11
Gurian, B. S., 25, 26, 27, 127

H

Hamasaki, 30
Hanawa, I., 46, 49
Hardin, R. C., et al., 124
Harding, R., 58, 75, 156, 157, 158
Hastings, A. B., 26
Hausler, H. R., et al., 139
Heath, H., *14–15*, 18, 84, 109, 122, 133, 137, *139–142*, *143–148*, 164
Hellström, B., 115, 121
Henkind, P., 3, 147, 148
Hubbard, R., 45
Hutchinson, B. T., 93, 94

This index is not intended to be comprehensive, but to indicate principal subject matters to the reader